PRAISE FOR
IMMUNOTHERAPY

"*Immunopatient* guides the reader through the new world of cancer immunotherapy... Anyone seeking to better understand immunotherapy will find this book to be compelling reading and a valuable roadmap."

—Gordon Freeman, PhD,
immunology researcher, Dana-Farber Cancer Institute;
Professor of Medicine, Harvard Medical School

"Written by a patient who has witnessed first-hand the evolution of cytokine therapy and the development of the new immune checkpoint inhibitors now widely advertised as a breakthrough in the management of advanced cancer, *Immunopatient* provides the reader with hope, inspiration, and a fact-based overview of the field of cancer immunotherapy."

—James Mier, MD,
Director of Laboratory Research, Biologics Therapy Program, Beth Israel-Deaconness Medical Center;
Associate Professor, Harvard Medical School

"In the cancer community we become family, confidantes, and co-conspirators against this disease that has us or our loved ones in its grasp. *Immunopatient* brings you into this world at a time when hopes have never been higher. Peter explains how and why in his gripping, heartfelt, deeply personal story. Read it."

—Robin Martinez,
Community Coordinator, SmartPatients.com

IMMUNOPATIENT

The New Frontier of
Curing Cancer

PETER ROONEY

Hatherleigh Press is committed to preserving and protecting the natural resources of the earth. Environmentally responsible and sustainable practices are embraced within the company's mission statement.

Visit us at www.hatherleighpress.com and register online for free offers, discounts, special events, and more.

Immunopatient

Library of Congress Cataloging-in-Publication Data is available.

ISBN: 978-1-57826-714-9

Printed in the United States

10 9 8 7 6 5 4 3 2 1

*To Katharina, my brave and kind wife,
I am eternally grateful for your
unstinting love and support.*

Contents

AUTHOR'S NOTE

Conversations in this book are depicted as accurately as possible, based upon memory, notes, and, in some cases, recordings. Some names and other identifying characteristics have been changed to protect the privacy of individuals.

Prologue
Rube Goldberg on a Drunken Bender, or How I Hope my Immune System Fights Cancer

Two days before Thanksgiving, Dr. James Mier called to tell me I had two new brain tumors.

He delivered the bad news as gently as possible—the tumors were extremely small, they could easily be zapped with high-dose radiation, and if all went well, I'd be cancer-free once again. But still, *two* new brain tumors? I had made so much progress fighting cancer over the last four years, but once again, reality was intruding on my plans for healing.

I did the best I could to take Dr. Mier at his word—he would know better than me, after all—but a question kept nagging at me. A question whose answer would have much further-reaching effects on my life and my treatment than I would have ever imagined.

Does my immune system work in the brain the same way it works in the rest of my body?

Dr. Mier said that, while he didn't know the answer to that question, he was inclined to think it didn't.

"I've always been a little doubtful," he explained. "If the immune system could get into the brain that easily, we'd all have

MS by now. But you shouldn't be discouraged. The good news is there's no evidence of cancer in the rest of your body, which could very well mean there aren't any cancer cells to travel to the brain and seed more tumors."

My reaction was, as you might expect, less than thrilled. "Cancer-free from the neck down is great and all," I said, "but I was hoping the news would be even better."

"I wouldn't be so quick to assume that the news won't be as good as all that in the future," Dr. Mier replied. "Remember, these small brain tumors are very receptive to radiation, and there may very well be an immune response. We just don't know yet."

I paused to think for a moment before asking, "Do you think Gordon Freeman would know?"

Dr. Mier paused as well before cautiously saying, "He might. If anybody would know, he would."

• • •

I'd first heard the name "Gordon Freeman" about a year earlier, while basking in the afterglow of a clean scan report.

"If you had to pick one person to thank for this," Dr. Mier remarked while reviewing the test results with me, "it would have to be Gordon Freeman at the Farber." Dr. Mier wore a tie and a plaid shirt beneath the traditional physician's uniform of a white laboratory coat, his name stitched in blue cursive on the left breast pocket.

"Who?" I asked.

"Gordon Freeman. He's your typical science geek. I get the sense that he doesn't realize how important his work is going to be, but people are already talking about a Nobel Prize for this new therapy of his. And not just for developing the therapeutics, but for elucidating the pathway where the immune system just dials itself down."

"Is he a pure researcher, or does he see patients?" I asked.

"He wouldn't know what a patient is," Dr. Mier replied as he signed off on the paperwork that gave the green light for the hospital pharmacy to create a dose of my experimental cancer treatment. "He's a hardcore molecular biologist."

Dr. Mier's eyes seemed to glow as he went on to describe exactly why pure research science is so crucial to the eventual development of drugs that may one day cure cancer. "You're working on something, by yourself, all the time with no idea whether it'll be important or not," he said. "Of course, a lot of hard work gets wasted or thrown into the waste basket because the basic idea is already incorrect. That's the nature of experimentation. But if you're fortunate enough to work on something that pans out in a major way, the value of that contribution is remarkable. And I think the Nobel committee may someday recognize that."

Dr. Mier's words resonated with me that day, and when I returned home I sent Freeman a holiday card in which I thanked him for his research. After all, it had led to a treatment I considered almost miraculous.

Almost a year later, with my original cancer still in remission, I sent Freeman an email, wondering whether he remembered the card and whether he might be willing to meet with me.

I now knew that Freeman was one of four scientists[1] with a background in immunology who collaborated *and* competed, preferring to zig together in their research pursuits where so many others were zagging, and who were now being credited for their unique insights—insights which were yielding a wave of promising new cancer treatments.

---

1 In addition to Freeman, the other scientists are: Lieping Chen of Yale University School of Medicine; Tasuku Honjo of Kyoto University School of Medicine; and Freeman's wife, Arlene Sharpe, of Harvard Medical School. They are beginning to gain more recognition both as a group and as individuals. For example, the four received the 2014 William B. Coley Award for Distinguished Research in Tumor Immunology from the Cancer Research Institute, which for several decades has advocated for using the body's own immune system to fight cancer. The award was for each scientist's research surrounding molecules, first discovered by Honjo, that have a curious function in the body's ridiculously complex immune system: they tell it to stand down after fighting off an infection.

Freeman quickly agreed to meet with me. It turned out he both remembered and appreciated my card from the year before. We settled on a date and time to meet in person, shortly after which I received the news about my two new brain tumors. Suddenly, what I had originally envisioned as a more detached conversation between a cancer survivor and a leading immunologist had become more urgent.

•   •   •

The poet Emily Dickinson calls hope "the thing with feathers," perhaps because the feeling itself can be so light and fleeting.

I was becoming increasingly worried by the information I was finding online about my prospective treatment options. What I read suggested that the various types of white blood cells that constitute the body's immune system don't easily pass through the blood-brain barrier.

I was quietly beginning to panic. Throughout my cancer treatments, one of the foundations of healing—for me, at least—was positive visualization. Picturing my body's white blood cells actively hunting down and killing cancer cells had become a vital mental exercise for me, one that helped me follow the concrete, scientifically-established path to remission and restored health. But that sense of focus and momentum was in danger of becoming unpinned as I pictured an impermeable locked gate somewhere at the base of my skull, keeping out a teeming swarm of frustrated T cells.

I was counting on Freeman to help me erase that scenario and replace it with a more hopeful image—ideally one that featured marauding T cells and melting cancer cells. Maybe he could offer some encouraging insights about how the immune system works in the brain and how it shrinks brain tumors like mine.

I know; it was a lot to hope for.

When I arrived, I found Freeman standing outside his office, smartly dressed in a navy blue cardigan sweater worn over a blue dress shirt and tucked into khaki pants. He offered me a slight smile and a handshake as he beckoned me into his office. Located on the fifth floor of the Dana-Farber Cancer Institute, his office was small yet cozy, with a tall window that offered a view of a cloud-shrouded dreary December day in Boston. A credenza stood nearby, crammed full with scientific journals.

After I sat down, placing my overcoat on a nearby chair, I asked him if he would allow me to record our conversation.

"I'm not sure what I'm going to do with all of this," I explained, "but I'm hoping to write a book about being a clinical trial patient. Getting things on tape means I don't have to try to take down every word, and hopefully I'll be more accurate when I try to write about the science."

Freeman hesitated for a moment before saying yes, he supposed that would be okay.

Whew, I thought. *Really glad he agreed to that one.*

As our conversation progressed, I soon found out that Freeman, much like other scientists at the top of their game, chose not to hide behind the esoteric vocabulary of his discipline. Throughout our talk, he demonstrated his skill at explaining the complex workings of the immune system in a way that interested "civilians" could understand. There certainly were moments when he'd say something that I only half-understood. But all it took was a hint of confusion on my part—a quizzical look, a furrowed brow—for Freeman to stop talking, consider for a moment, and come up with a better way to explain it.

It was just such a bewildered expression that prompted Freeman to reach for his favorite metaphor to describe the complex and convoluted workings of the immune system. "We're not talking about intelligent design here," he said. "It's more like 'Rube Goldberg[2] on a Drunken Bender.'"

---

2 This Rube Goldberg analogy will be familiar to some, but not all. Since 1932, Webster's has considered "Rube Goldberg" to be an adjective, referring to doing something simple in a very complicated way. The term derives from a popular cartoon panel that appeared in newspapers during the 1920s and 1930s. Penned by Rube Goldberg, an engineer turned Pulitzer Prize-winning cartoonist, the cartoons depicted schematics dreamed up by one of his characters, Professor Lucifer Gorgonzola Butts, for machines that used not only belts, pulleys and levers, but also animals, auto bumpers, buckets, shoes,

I couldn't help laughing, startled at the vivid chaos such an image brings to mind.

"The reason I say that," Freeman continued, "is because the immune system is under continual assault by different infectious diseases. Each of them tries to invade, overcome, or get around the immune system in a different way. So, if you try to attack the measles virus using just one method, measles will always be quicker and more nimble. It'll learn to evade a single attack. On the other hand, if you attack the measles virus from ten different directions, measles might be able to evade one or two of those attacks, but the other eight will get it."

Freeman's insight into the immune system's insane complexity is hard-earned. His curriculum vitae (or CV) shows not only the typical fare—things like job titles, peer reviewed papers authored, honors received, research grants awarded, and degrees earned—but also included a section for "patents awarded." There were 48 in total at last count. His first came in 1992, and twenty-two patents were awarded between 2000 and 2006. This was when much of the basic research that has led to the new wave of immunotherapy drugs, recently approved by the FDA, was conducted.

By the time I met with Freeman, I was fairly familiar with the science behind the experimental cancer treatment that I had been receiving for the last fourteen months. At the time, I was in a Phase 1 clinical trial at Beth Israel Deaconess Medical Center in

---

paddles, and even canary cages. Goldberg depicted these contraptions with artistic flair in black pen and ink drawings, accompanied by clever captions, including this one for "closing a window if it starts to rain while you're away":

Pet bull frog, A, homesick for water, hears rainstorm and jumps for joy, pulling string, B, which opens catch, C, and releases hot water bag, D, allowing it to slide under chair, E. Heat raises yeast, F, lifting disc, G, which causes hook, H, to release spring, I. Toy automobile bumper, J, socks monkey, K, in the neck putting him down for the count on table, L. He staggers to his feet and slips on banana peel, M. He instinctively reaches for flying rings, N, to avoid further disaster and his weight pulls rope, O, closing window, P, stopping the rain from leaking through on the family downstairs and thinning their soup.

Boston that combined two recently developed immune therapy treatments. One of them, called ipilimumab and marketed under the brand name Yervoy, had received FDA approval in 2011. The other drug was called nivolumab, brand name Opdivo, referred to by medical staff at Beth Israel as PD-1. (My shorthand for the two is ipi and nivo.) After signing a clinical trial consent form that listed over fifty-three pages of side effects noted in the trial thus far, I had been given both drugs for the first three months and nivo alone since then. Every two weeks, the drug dosage was calibrated to my body weight and given to me through an IV line, which dripped the drugs into my bloodstream over the course of an hour.

As Dr. Mier had explained it to me, the treatment kept my T cells, a type of white blood cell the body uses to fight off infection, from being turned off. This gives the cells more time to hunt down and kill the cancer cells in my body. It seemed to be a simple enough concept; I wondered why it had taken so long to discover the treatment.

The reason, as it turned out, was because scientists still have so much to discover about the molecular workings of the immune system. Freeman began studying the immune system as a doctoral student at Harvard in the 1970s, his studies eventually leading him to a Ph.D. in microbiology and molecular genetics in 1979. Two post-doctoral fellowships followed, both at the Dana-Farber Cancer Institute. He was matter-of-fact about what led him to immunology, saying that it was an "opportune" time to dive into the field, especially for someone with a personality like his, which he described as, "very curious, probably shy. Retiring, ethereal; I'm a discoverer, I'm not a tremendous political fighter. I don't like conflict. I like peace and quiet."

And it seems he made his choice wisely. The Farber, as he often calls it, has pretty much left him alone over the years, content to see him churning out papers, reeling in grants, and plugging away in his quest to better understand the immune system and the different types of white blood cells that comprise its fighting force, especially the T cells responsible for combatting diseases as varied as cancer and AIDS.

In the course of becoming what he calls a "competent molecular biologist" during his post-doctoral years, he decided that the opportune thing to do was to "clone a gene," and focused his efforts on duplicating a gene called B7. This molecule had been discovered by Arnie Freedman and Freeman while both were post-docs in Lee Nadler's lab at the Dana-Farber, during which time they established that the B7 molecule strongly stimulated immune responses by activating T cells.

"It was sending an important signal," Freeman explained. "But the other thing that was surprising was that the B7 molecule had *two* receptors; the other receptor, which is called CTLA-4, actually turned *off* the immune response."

Even as Freeman was working to clone the B7 gene, the Human Genome Project was being launched in a massive bid to assemble a complete transcription of the tremendously complex genetic blueprint for building a human being.

"Suddenly, instead of cloning one gene at a time, you had 25,000 to look at," Freeman said. Their single B7 molecule had become an entire family of related B7 molecules. "We found two more molecules called PD-L1 and PD-L2. Then, with Clive Wood at the Genetics Institute, we showed that a molecule called PD-1 was the receptor that bound to PD-L1 and PD-L2.

"You could say one of the molecules is a key and the other is a lock—they fit into each other," Freeman said. "So, if you want to make a drug which blocks something, what you need to do is block the key from going into the hole. If you made a blocker which binds to the part of the key that fits in your hand—the part that doesn't interact with the lock at any point—it's not going to prevent anything from happening. So our findings defined what the lock and key relationship was, *and* what its function was, which was how we showed that it inhibited immune responses."

Freeman paused for a moment to make sure I was still following him—I was, if only barely—and then continued. "This finding was a surprise, because most things are expected to increase the immune response. It was somewhat unexpected to find there were molecules that shut it down."

Freeman and his collaborators began pursuing a counterintuitive notion—that the mission to cure cancer and other chronic diseases could perhaps be achieved by understanding how white blood cells such as T cells and natural killer (NK) cells were turned off, rather than how they were stimulated.

What fascinated me as I tried to visualize the experimental treatment coursing through my veins (and hopefully making its way into my brain, as well) was how Freeman and his colleagues had arrived at these particular genes to study.

"Certainly, computer analysis was essential in our discovery," Freeman said when I asked him about it. "We couldn't look at and compare 25,000 things without the rapid processing capacity of a computer. But even that just gave us hints and suggestions. It didn't prove anything. So we then had to make the molecules and make the antibodies and do the experiments in the test tubes and in mice to show just what the molecules do."

Curing cancer in mice using immune therapy is one thing; doing so in humans is quite another. "It's been sort of promised for a long time, and different laboratories *have* cured cancer in a mouse," Freeman said. "But none of them translated to a successful human therapy; the treatments either didn't work in people or they were too dangerous. But now that's changed."

What also changed was the willingness of Freeman and other immunologists to look at the puzzle of curing cancer in a new way, by focusing on what turns *off* the immune system, and then trying to devise ways to prevent that from happening.

"The old idea was always 'stimulate the immune response to make it stronger,'" Freeman explained. "Vaccination is a great example of this, and is wonderfully successful at preventing, say, smallpox, because your body has never seen smallpox before—you can make an antibody against it when you're vaccinated. What we realize now is that cancer is a chronic disease. When you go into your doctor's office because of how you're feeling and get a diagnosis of cancer, it's not something that just happened. It's been a five, ten, or twenty year development. Throughout that period, your immune system has been looking at the cancer and trying to fight it off. When it succeeds, you don't go to the doctor's office; you never experienced any problems from it. But when the immune system fails, it's because the cancer has learned to evade the immune system. That's when it becomes a real problem.

"What we've since learned is that the immune system has multiple ways to turn off its immune response, one of which is the expression of the PD-L1 molecule. When expressed, PD-L1 basically acts as a shield or a cloak on the tumor and keeps the immune system from attacking it successfully."

For some time, I'd noticed Freeman occasionally glancing at a clear glass rectangular box mounted on a platform on his desk. Suspended inside the glass appeared to be two wispy strands.

"Is that a model of the PD-1 molecule, by chance?" I asked.

"It is indeed," he said with an eager grin, reaching over to grab it. "You can see that the PDL-1 fits into this surface right here on the PD-1. That 'lock and key' interaction turns off the PD-1, which then shuts down the immune response, allowing the cancer to grow. The drugs are basically things that bind or cover over either the lock or the key. You can bind to the PD-1 side, or the PD-L1 side; both will work."

Freeman didn't develop the drug itself. That task was taken on by Alan Korman and Nils Longren (among others), scientists at Medarex, a biotechnology company that was acquired by Bristol-Myers Squibb for $2.4 billion in 2009. Already, Korman and Longren had successfully converted the B7 molecule's CTLA-4 mechanism discovered by Freeman and his team into an antibody, which eventually became the ipi (or Yervoy) currently residing-- and hopefully working--in my system.

Since then, several immune therapy cancer treatments that modulate T-cells have entered clinical trials. Bristol-Myers Squibb's Yervoy (ipilimumab) is based on the CTLA-4 mechanism and was approved by the FDA in 2011 for metastatic melanoma. Another Bristol-Myers Squibb product, Opdivo (nivolumab), which is based on blocking PD-1, was given FDA approval in December 2014 for the treatment of advanced melanoma and squamous non-small cell lung cancer, and has also been approved for use in Japan and Europe. Meanwhile, Merck & Co.'s Keytruda (pembrolizumab) surprised many pharmaceutical industry observers by being the first PD-1 drug approved by the FDA in the United States, receiving the green light in September 2014.

While analysts predict that these drugs will be expensive, with treatment courses costing $100,000 or more, they are also likely to be pervasive, with experts like Freeman predicting that immune therapies will supplant chemotherapy as a first line cancer treatment within five to ten years.

Exactly how much money will come to Freeman and Dana-Farber as a result of nivolumab's development remains to be seen, and will be determined by royalty rates negotiated by Dana-Farber on the patent claims that pertain to the development of nivolumab and other immune therapies that draw upon Freeman's work.

Financial benefits notwithstanding, Freeman says his true passion remains his work to better understand the immune system so that cancer and other chronic diseases like hepatitis and AIDS can be conquered (or at least tamed).

Curious, I asked whether Freeman felt vindicated in his decades-long quest to better understand the molecular machinations of the immune system and to use such understanding to fight disease. He smiled broadly and said, "Absolutely."

"Why is that?" I asked.

"Five years ago, if I said I was doing immunotherapy in cancer, the response would have been, 'It's a nice idea, but it's not in your doctor's office.' For a long time, immunotherapy was a nice idea, but not successful. Ipi and nivo have really brought some success. It feels good because it shows that the ideas you've championed for so long are working. You really *can* successfully treat cancer if you can block the cancer from inhibiting the immune response."

Since the initial research that led to the development of nivolumab and other PD-1-based treatments, Freeman and others have discovered that inhibition by PD-1 is a common occurrence in the body's immune system, and that certain chronic diseases such as tuberculosis, malaria, hepatitis C, and AIDS cause T cells to become laden with PD-1 molecules, each of them an off switch waiting to be flipped.

"In all of these diseases, the immune system tries to fight the disease, doesn't succeed, and then the immune system just goes quiet," Freeman said. "It tunes down. It keeps attacking, but only moderately. It finds a balance.

"Say you have hepatitis. Your body doesn't want to attack it so strongly that it destroys the liver, because you can't live without a liver. So, you attack and keep the virus low, but you don't burn it out.

"What we've also realized is that in all these chronic infections, the T cells that are attacking the disease have lots of PD-1 molecules on them. They're always susceptible to being turned off by PD-L1. And cancer, we now recognize, is like a chronic disease. It's not like a T cell coming across a tumor is seeing it for the first time. It's been there 100 times in the last ten years."

• • •

This all sounded very encouraging, yet there was still the issue of the brain and whether there was any reason to believe my body's T cells, their off switches shielded to extend their life spans, could find their way into my brain.

"What kind of treatment are you on, by the way?" Freeman asked, taking a break from his explanation.

I quickly described my treatment and the clinical trial's parameters: I had been on the trial since July 2013, and I was among the half of about 130 patients in the trial who had received a lower dose of ipi, one milligram per kilogram of body weight, compared to three milligrams per kilogram for the other half. We were all receiving a nivo dose of three milligrams per kilogram.

"I got the results of my last scans after you and I set up our meeting," I told Freeman. "It was good news from the neck down, but there are two new small tumors in the brain. I'm happy about everything, but obviously I'm worried about what's going on upstairs. There's also a little concern about some swelling they're seeing on a spot I had treated about two years ago. Tomorrow I go in for a Cyberknife treatment to zap the two spots on the brain."

I shifted nervously in my seat. "I guess that leads me to my current dilemma, which I see as a roadblock on my path to healing. I'm very much interested in the science of my treatment, but I've also been reading about the connection between the mind and the body, the power of the placebo effect, things like that."

I paused to see whether he was rolling his eyes yet. He wasn't, which was encouraging, so I continued. "Where I've hit a bit of a dead end is that so much of what I'm reading suggests that the immune system doesn't really penetrate the blood-brain barrier. That's a good thing, I guess, because the cells in the brain are so densely packed that you'd see a lot of swelling if there were a lot of white blood cells up there. So I'm wondering if you could tell me a little about the immune system and whether it works in the brain."

Left unsaid but hopefully understood was my real question: *Is there any reason to hope my immune system can fight cancer in the brain?*

"Basically," Freeman began, "the blood vessels of the brain have a tighter fit than blood vessels in, say, your legs. So they *can* keep *drugs* from getting in and out. But *white blood cells* can still get in and out. For instance, the brain cancer that scientists conduct the most research on is glioblastoma. If you start glioblastoma in a mouse brain and treat it with CTLA-4 and PD-1, the tumor gets attacked and eliminated. So immune cells *can* attack brain tumors. In fact, I think people are now starting to de-emphasize just how tight the blood brain barrier is against T cell attack."

"That's great," I said. "I'm looking for something to be hopeful about."

"You're an example of a combination therapy," he replied. "Nivo plus ipi. The good thing about that is it's the most successful combination we've seen so far. But we're also seeing that many things can work with PD-1 to make the response rate even higher, including other immunological drugs, certain chemotherapies, and even radiation."

This gave me some pause. During the course of fighting my cancer, I had come to the grim realization that all cancer treatments extract their toll. Radiation may kill cancer cells, but it can also encourage mutations that lead to cancer later on. Xgeva, a drug I took to help rebuild radiated bone in my left humerus and right femur, can also cause necrosis in jawbones. Chemotherapy, in the form of an infusion or pill, has very serious side effects as well, but so far I had not needed to endure them.

"I'm getting radiation tomorrow," I told him. "It's called a Cyberknife, but it's really a high dose of focused radiation on those two spots."

He nodded and offered some more perspective from the cutting edge of cancer research. "Five years ago, I would have said radiation just kills cells directly," he said. "But it's since become clear that radiation has a lot of effects on the immune system, as well. In a mouse, if you radiate a tumor in the arm, you can spark an immune activation which will attack a tumor in, say, the liver. Radiation and PD-1 can also synergize and work together to attack cancer cells all over the body."

"In the brain, as well?" I asked.

He nodded. "Again, I think the immune system accesses the brain. The worry isn't that it can't access the brain; it's more that if you get brain swelling, do you have to treat with steroids to dampen things down?"

He quickly added a qualifier: "Remember, I'm not a physician, so don't take any of this as medical fact."

"Don't worry about that," I replied. "But I still really appreciate the insight. And I really appreciate your work on all of this, and for sticking with it for so long."

I stood up to leave, but before heading out, I asked whether I could take some photos of him at his desk. He graciously agreed, and between shots he stressed how quickly the field of immunotherapy is evolving and how promising the new treatments seem to be, primarily because their application allows for multiple angles of treatment approach.

"The weakness of classic chemotherapy is that it's focused on one target," he said. "It can work initially, but the tumor learns to evade the attack. Ten months later, the chemotherapy doesn't work any longer. The difference with immunotherapy is that it lets the immune system attack the cancer eight or ten different ways. It's harder for the tumor to learn to evade lots of different ways of attack."

He offered a mild-mannered smile. "I sort of think of it as attacking with a machine gun rather than a single shooter."

As I exited his office, a number of young Dana-Farber employees just outside Freeman's door glanced up at me from their computer workstations. I briefly wondered how much of our conversation they had heard. Already I was feeling more optimistic about the future. I knew that my outward appearance betrayed no evidence of the cancer in my body, which was now confined to only a few small spots in my brain. And if science, my mind, and my body had anything to say about it, even those would be gone soon enough.

PART I
Confronting and Coping

1 Slip-Sliding Away

If you've ever lost control of your car, you know that you experience every micro-second in slow motion. That's exactly what happened to me one cold grey morning in late February 2011, when I hit a patch of ice entering a roundabout, just after the car ahead of me did the same.

As I jerked my steering wheel to avoid a collision, a scaring jolt of pain in my upper left arm caused me to gasp. I struggled to concentrate on the two sliding cars while my brain worked overtime to register the extreme pain I was feeling in my arm. I continued my slow-motion slide, straightened out the steering wheel with my right hand, and just managed to miss the other vehicle.

While I was certainly shaken up and considered getting out to check on the other driver, since there'd been no collision and my pain was not subsiding, I instead continued on my way to work.

I parked at Amherst College, climbed the three flights of marble stairs in the old library building that had been converted to serve as classrooms and offices, walked into my office, turned on my computer, and sat down at my desk. As I gingerly tried to lift my left arm to my desktop, I found I couldn't do so without feeling a stab of intense pain.

That's not good, I thought. *Not good at all. I hope I can still go on that trip.*

In less than two weeks, my wife Katharina and I were leaving for Belize to celebrate our twenty-fifth wedding anniversary.

It was to be the honeymoon trip we couldn't afford when we married in Vienna in 1986, as twenty-one-year-old students with so much to learn about life but who nevertheless knew that we loved each other.

I wanted to make sure I had this nagging injury looked at and taken care of before our trip, even if it meant wearing a sling or a brace. I'd been seeing a physical therapist for several weeks to deal with discomfort in my shoulder and upper arm. I thought the pain was a result of my exercise routine—one that included swimming, push-ups, and sets of chin-ups. Teingo West, my physical therapist, had me doing various range-of-motion exercises, and I'd seemed to making steady progress...until the ice slide and my steering wheel jerk, that is.

Teingo will sort it out. He'll just give me some new exercises, and I'll start doing them. I've got almost two weeks to get better—no problem!

• • •

Later that day at his clinic, West was puzzled that I was unable to lift my left arm much at all, either to the side or over my head. A muscular man from Ghana with a decidedly pleasant manner, West was especially struck by how much pain I felt and how little resistance I could offer when he pushed against my arm.

"I'm not sure what it could be," he finally said, "but if it doesn't get better by Thursday, you should go see an orthopedic surgeon." Hardly the assessment I'd been hoping for.

I can't wait that long doing nothing, I thought. *If I broke something, I want to get it treated* now. *Better to nip a small problem in the bud before it becomes a bigger problem.* I moved my left arm and once again let out a gasp of pain. *Because I can feel right now that things are not going to get better by doing nothing.*

So I called the office of my primary care doctor, Richard Wu, and his assistant scheduled me for an appointment the next day. It was Dr. Wu who had written the order for my physical therapy about four weeks earlier, so he was somewhat familiar with my situation.

I had picked Dr. Wu to be my primary care doctor soon after starting my job as Amherst College's Director of Public Affairs in the fall of 2008, but an active lifestyle and a generally clean bill of health meant I hadn't seen him too much in the nearly five years since then. That said, I'd always liked his laid-back demeanor and the low-key way he'd encouraged me to lose about fifteen pounds a couple of years earlier, after he observed that my blood pressure and cholesterol level were creeping into the high range.

Dr. Wu's medical practice was housed in a low-slung brick building that shared space with the town newspaper. It was near the University of Massachusetts campus, located across the street from an outpost of Cooley Dickinson Hospital that included a blood lab and a radiology department. The waiting room was about three-quarters full that morning, mostly older patients reading magazines. I took my place among them, flipping nervously through the pages of *Sports Illustrated* until my name was called.

A nurse's assistant ushered me into an examining room. Inside, she checked my blood pressure and other vital signs before instructing me to strip to my t-shirt and undershorts and wait for the doctor. Given the immobility of my left arm, this took some doing and was anything but painless.

After about five minutes of waiting, there was a short rap on the door of the examining room and Dr. Wu entered.

"So, your left arm is still giving you trouble," he said, reading from a laptop that he held in the crook of his arm. "And...you had an accident recently?"

Okay, I thought to myself. *You're on. Tell him about the accident and he'll fix you up. That's what doctors do.*

I recounted the mishap, and he asked whether I could lift my arm over my head. I gave my arm a feeble lift until the pain in my upper arm told me to stop.

"Not even close," I replied.

"So we'll need to order an x-ray," he noted. "It's probably just a muscle tear, so the x-ray won't see anything, but the HMO won't approve an MRI without it."

I walked across the street to the x-ray lab, where they took the pictures of my shoulder. My arm was too sore for me to move it much, so they had to position it on the plates. Then it was back to my office to await the results.

I tried to spend the time productively, tending to a few projects. One of them was publicizing a reading honoring the 90th birthday of Richard Wilbur, the celebrated American poet and Amherst College lecturer. Wilbur had served in the infantry during World War II and his poems had appeared in *The New Yorker* for decades, during which he had twice been awarded the Pulitzer Prize for poetry. At 90, Wilbur still stood taller than my 6'3" and carried his solid mass up and down the stairs of Converse Hall twice each week with slow yet vibrant grace as he made his way to teach his poetry seminar.

A literary lion in his 90s, and he still plays tennis, I mused from my desk. *I wonder if he dyes his hair, though. He'd be a true medical marvel if that brown hair was natural.*

It was cold and slushy outside, so I stayed inside for my lunchtime workout. As my legs scissored back and forth on the elliptical machine at the college's gym, I tried to gauge the pain in my left arm.

Is it worse or better than last week? I asked myself. With my left hand, I gripped the handles of the elliptical, which moved back and forth in sync with the two rimmed platforms that supported my feet. *Last week I could do this.* My arm pumped with the handle, and every time it extended, pain shot through my bone.

So I kept my left arm close at my side, careful not to exceed its range. I still wasn't too worried; I'd had some shoulder pain off and on for the last few months, but I was forty-six—surely these were simply the aches and pains of middle age. So for the next forty-five minutes, I focused solely on working up a sweat and tried to ignore the discomfort that lingered at the edge of my mind.

I finished my post-workout shower and carefully dressed in the college's locker room. I was taking care not to tweak my arm as I threaded it through my sleeve when I noticed I had two voicemails from Dr. Wu's office.

"Peter," he said when I finally reached him, "the radiologist very clearly saw a bone lesion in your left humerus. You need to come in tomorrow and get a CT scan and bone scan."

Well…that's not exactly good news, is it?

"A lesion?" I asked, trying to sound unconcerned. "What's that all about?"

"We don't know exactly what it is, but the radiologist definitely sees something on the bone," he replied, and wouldn't say anything more about it.

And so the next day Katharina and I drove to Cooley Dickinson Hospital in Northampton. My state of mind wasn't what I would call great; I had spent the evening searching for information on bone lesions online, and the results didn't make for a good night's sleep. I was worried, but still hopeful that my scans would clear things up. After all, x-rays weren't always accurate.

A CT scan (where CT stands for "computed tomography") takes numerous x-rays of the body's internal organs, creating visual slices that radiologists can then examine. In my case, the scanner would be taking images of my chest, pelvis, and abdomen, while the bone scanner checked for bone density and construction.

The bone scan required only a radioactive tracer injection to enhance resolution. For the CT scan, however, Katharina watched as I drank a vile-tasting barium-laced concoction followed by an injection of contrast dye just before passing beneath the donut-shaped scanning machine.

It was hardly what I would call pleasant. But then, over the next several years I would become all too familiar with both of these unpleasant procedures, along with the unsettling, nerve-wracking anxiety that quickly settles in while awaiting one's results.

2 Everything Changes

I arrived for my appointment with Dr. Wu the next morning at 10:30 am sharp, and this time I didn't have to wait. The receptionist ushered me into the examining room, and I spent the next couple minutes trying to calm my racing thoughts before a brief rap on the door announced the doctor's arrival.

Whippet-thin and looking anxious, Dr. Wu plunged right into the bad news.

"That lesion on your left arm, it's actually cancer," he said, nodding to himself nervously. "Kidney cancer, or renal cell cancer; it's one of the most common cancers that goes to bone."

The words echoed in my head. I felt very alone all of a sudden, which was partially my fault. I had told Katharina that she didn't need to make the trip with me, that I would be perfectly happy to patch her into my appointment with Dr. Wu using my phone.

I knew it was time to bring her into the conversation. I dialed her number and she picked up after the first ring.

"Hello?" Katharina's voice sounded worried and very, very far away.

"Hi Katharina, it's Peter. I'm here with Dr. Wu, so you can listen in on the conversation." "That would be nice, thank you." She sounded like she was struggling to keep her voice even.

Dr. Wu continued. "Katharina, I just told Peter that the lesion on his left arm is connected to kidney cancer, one that has metastasized from the kidney to the left arm." Without pausing for a reply, he went on, "The first thing to do is to move forward with an orthopedic appointment. The radiologist tells me Peter's left arm is so fragile that even routine activities could cause the arm to fracture."

Dr. Wu sat at down at his desk and, with a few taps at his keyboard, brought up the results of my scans.

"Here's what we know from the CT scan of the chest, abdomen, and pelvis. The primary lesion is on the kidney, and the radiologist says it looks like a classic kidney cancer lesion. It's 7.1 centimeters, something like 2 inches by 3 inches."

"A lesion is a tumor?" I asked, still working to process everything I was being told.

The doctor nodded. "The bone scan also found a second bony lesion located in the right femur—the long bone of the leg. It doesn't sound as though the lesion on the right femur is as severe as the lesion on the left humerus, but obviously Dr. Fallon—he's the orthopedic surgeon —will need to consider whether or not both lesions require a procedure."

Dr. Wu paused for a moment, collecting his thoughts. This was obviously a difficult conversation for him.

"The two other doctors who would be involved with your case would be a urologist—because if the primary tumor is in the kidney or the kidney itself needs to be removed, it's a urologist who'll perform that procedure—and an oncologist, as they're the ones who manage the radiation and any resulting chemotherapy."

I didn't have much to say. This was a lot of information coming at me all at once, and I could only think, *How is someone who has been diagnosed with cancer supposed to react? Should I scream? Should I cry? Should I show any emotion at all?*

I managed to nod and maintain eye contact with Dr. Wu. I was depending on him to keep talking and explaining while I struggled to absorb his words and control the dread that was flooding my brain.

"Kidney cancer tends to present in people who are a lot older than forty-six, that's for sure," he was saying, looking puzzled. "Though I do actually have a different patient in his thirties who was diagnosed with kidney cancer within the last six months. They did a partial kidney resection, and he seems to be doing okay. I would like to send you to the same urologist that he worked with; both he and his wife felt they received very good, compassionate treatment."

There—the urologist and the patient who'd been through kidney cancer. That was a concrete step to jump onto, a bit of good news to focus on.

"So this urologist—is he around here?" I asked.

Dr. Wu nodded. "Florence," he said, referring to a small town near Northampton.

I decided to ask the big question. "And as far as cancers go… how bad or good is the prognosis?"

"It spans the range," he replied. "My uncle was diagnosed with kidney cancer, as a matter of fact. That was…probably four or five years ago now, and he's doing pretty well."

So that was good news. But I was still worried about the fact that the cancer was in my bones now, too. That couldn't be good.

"Do the bony lesions indicate whether this is on the worse end of the spectrum?"

"Well, it means that the cancer's left the kidney itself," he said, clearly unhappy. "That definitely implies a more severe case – Stage IV, or metastatic cancer in other words. So I'll set up the referral to the specialists I mentioned."

He glanced at his computer and then back at me. "Any other questions off the top of your head?"

I had plenty, but they were all half-formed and panicky: *Will I need chemotherapy? Can I beat this cancer? Can I keep on working?*

And the worst of the lot: *Am I going to die soon?*

I decided to ask something that was more focused on the here-and-now. "Well," I began, "I know this may seem real short-term in the grand scheme of things, but my wife and I were planning a trip to Belize. What are the chances I could still go?"

Not very high, as it turned out. "Your arm could easily fracture just by performing simple activities," Dr. Wu cautioned. "Dr. Fallon will probably want to fix that as soon as possible. It's just not realistic to consider going on that trip."

"Dr. Fallon is the orthopedic surgeon, right?" I asked. "What would he be doing?"

"Typically, the orthopedic surgeon would put in a metal rod to stabilize that bone," Dr. Wu said. "I really couldn't say exactly when, but based on what the radiologist said, being out of the country and away from top-rated medical facilities would be too risky for such a weak arm."

I felt my future slipping away from me. Everything was changing, and quickly. I felt like I had just been strapped into the scariest roller-coaster ride imaginable, one that goes through dark tunnels, stomach-churning drops, and body-twisting corkscrews with no end in sight.

"So what happens now?" I asked, suddenly exhausted. "Should I start making arrangements to take a medical leave from work, or go on disability?"

"It's pretty likely you'll need to go on some sort of disability," Dr. Wu agreed. "That arm surgery's going to be a pretty big procedure, and while I'm not a urologist, and I don't know if they would plan on removing part or all of your kidney. Either way, that's a pretty big surgery, too."

Finally, I asked the question that had been lurking in my mind as the news settled in.

"What's the mortality rate for kidney cancer?"

"Well, the best person to ask that would be either the urologist or the oncologist," Dr. Wu said, sidestepping the question. "That's their field. I wouldn't want to misquote and give you a prognosis that was either unfairly horrible or falsely hopeful."

"Right," I said, not happy with the answer but unwilling to press any further.

"Did you have any other questions, or anything you want repeated?" Dr. Wu asked.

Coming through on the speaker phone, Katharina weighed in: "The cancer. Is it malignant at this point?"

Dr. Wu replied, "For a definitive diagnosis you'd need tissue for a biopsy. And there's a fair chance that will still happen. On the other hand, the radiologist indicated this is a pretty classic case. There wasn't a hint of doubt in his mind when he described his findings."

"We, umm, we have a friend who passed away from kidney cancer," Katharina said, having trouble finishing the sentence. "This...sounds really serious."

"It *is* serious," Dr. Wu replied. "That's why we want to coordinate things and get underway as quickly as possible. I'll get to work immediately on lining up the necessary appointments for Peter."

"Peter?" she asked. "Can I speak to you?"

I picked up the phone, turning it off speaker for the moment.

"What do you want me to do?" she asked. "Do you want me to drive down and meet you?"

"No, that's all right," I said. "I think I'll just come home. Though maybe I should go back to work and let my boss know what's going on."

"You could do that if you wanted to," Dr. Wu said. "Or you could just go home and not worry about the work situation right now. Workplaces tend to be pretty understanding about serious illness. You might want to go home instead and try to compose yourself over the weekend. You know...try to mentally prepare yourself for the tough times ahead."

"You have a point," I admitted. "I think I'll do just that." I stood up from the examining table and began to get dressed.

"Boy," Dr. Wu said. "When you came in on Tuesday, I was really hoping it would just be an orthopedic situation."

"Me, too," I said. As I prepared to leave, my thoughts turned to a question that would later surface again and again. "I'm just thinking about whether this could all have been caught any earlier."

"Well, you weren't symptomatic earlier," Dr. Wu mused. "In fact, perhaps jerking the wheel was actually a good thing. It could have been another month or two or three if that didn't happen."

My head was still spinning as I turned to leave. I tried to thank Dr. Wu for his time, but nothing coherent came out of my mouth.

"Well," I finally managed, "there's a lot of information here for me to process. My life has changed, obviously."

"Yeah," Dr. Wu agreed. "You're going to be busy with appointments in the immediate future with the people you really need to see."

And how do I know if they're the right people to be treating me? I wondered. *And how do I ask that without sounding snobby and elitist?*

"If I get people telling me 'you should go to this person' or 'you should go to Boston,'" I began, "how do I go about evaluating the quality of the care and the specialist?"

"I think starting with local specialists is a good idea, no matter what you end up deciding to do," he replied. "I wouldn't be able to say whether or not a certain specialist in Boston was the person to see or not, but physicians in Boston would. And the local specialists aren't bad, either.

"We're going to go through this process together," he added as he shook my hand and turned to leave the examining room. "We'll get those appointments scheduled for you next week and I'll keep watching your case."

He closed the door, and I was all but alone in the room, save for Katharina still on the line.

"Katharina, it's just us again," I said. "How are you feeling?"

"I'm feeling okay, Peter. How are you?"

"I'm okay, too. I'm actually looking forward to the drive home. I can start thinking about my situation, and how we tell the boys about this. I'll see you in about an hour."

"Drive safe," she said. "I love you. We'll get through this together."

"I know we will," I said.

Though I couldn't see how.

3 Sinking In

*L*ife's a bitch and then you die.

I had first heard that phrase as a teenager, and I remember responding with a knowing, adolescent nod, embracing the sentiment and realizing then, as now, that for most people on this planet, life *is* a struggle and death *does* come to all.

If people weren't confronting health issues like mine, they were worried about keeping their jobs, or had already lost them, or had their homes foreclosed on, or lost unemployment benefits before they had found work elsewhere, or found themselves settling for dead-end jobs.

Even in nature, adversity was the order of the day. Hatchling birds, pecking slime-covered beaks through egg encasings, desperately open their mouths for food that may never come. A few tiny sea turtles crawl from their eggs towards the sea, only to be eaten by birds and other predators before they get there.

As for humans, hard-wired to seek survival though we are, we can't help but assess the odds of success and survival in any given situation, part of an intuitive calculation of whether a fight is worth fighting.

Whether there is reason for hope.

Everyone deals with adversity, illness, and death. In the U.S. alone, half of all men and one-third of all individuals will develop cancer during their lifetimes. People are suffering everywhere in almost unimaginable ways.

So went my thoughts, still reeling from receiving what could well be my death sentence. Suddenly, a line from an old country song wafted through my brain: "Don't tell me your troubles. I got troubles of my own."

True enough. But they are my *troubles, and no one is going to solve them but me.*

So I decided to drive back to the office where I had left my laptop and see whether I could uncover any signs of hope for the battle I was about to face.

I walked by Maryann, our office's administrative assistant, being careful to avoid eye contact. I was still digesting the news of my cancer diagnosis, and didn't trust myself to be able to hold it together.

In my office, sitting down at the computer I'd left on, I couldn't resist a quick search for the two terms that had been swimming around in my brain: "renal cancer" and "bone lesion."

I soon found myself at bonetumor.org, where I was treated to the following:

> *"Renal cell cancers rank as the approximately sixth most common site of origin of metastatic deposits in the skeleton. Although the number of cases of this cancer is proportionally small, the tumor has a high avidity for bone and thus creates relatively large numbers of bone lesions. Patients may have no other manifestation of cancer other than their painful bone lesion. Because the primary tumor can grow fairly large without creating local symptoms such as flank pain or a mass in the abdomen, kidney cancer often presents only when a metastasis develops. When a patient has a metastasis and no site of origin can be found (a metastasis of unknown origin) the most likely site is the lung or kidney.*
>
> *Patients are usually over 40, and the average age is around 55. Pain is the most common presenting symptom. Pathological fracture rarely occurs without a history of a few weeks or months of increasingly severe pain.*
>
> *In some cases, patients will try to ignore or deny the symptoms.*

Denial certainly described me. I had been dealing with a sore shoulder for months and had been unwilling to scale back my physical activities, even though sleeping and even dressing myself was becoming increasingly difficult. On the weekend before my slide on the ice, I had not only gone cross-country skiing, but downhill skiing, as well. Sure, I felt twinges of pain when I planted my left ski pole, and I couldn't close my ski boots buckles with my left hand because of pain in my upper arm. I wrote it all off as old age or sore muscles.

I went to the next search result, a site maintained by the American Academy of Orthopedic Surgeons, which offered the following perspective:

> *The most common cancers that arise from organs and spread to bone include Breast, Lung, Thyroid, Kidney and Prostate. Metastatic Bone Disease (MBD) causes pain in the area of spread, damages and weakens bone, and puts the patient at a greater risk for broken bones. It can make it hard to participate in daily activities. The biggest concern for patients with MBD is the general loss in quality of life.*

The page finished with a carefully worded sentence, clearly intended to be neither encouraging nor discouraging:

> *Advances in surgical techniques as well as radiation and medical therapies have significantly improved the quality of life for the individual suffering from cancer that has spread to the skeleton from its site of origin. Treatment options for MBD are based upon how much the cancer has spread, which bones are affected, and how severe the bone damage.*

•   •   •

I had read enough; it was time to go home. Before turning off my computer, I sent my boss, Susan Pikor, a brief email update, ending with, "Any thoughts on specialists would be appreciated. I am meeting with an orthopedic surgeon and urologist on Monday. 7.1 cm tumor in right kidney; decent sized lesion in left arm (humerus); another small lesion identified in right femur."

She called me as I was sliding my laptop into my briefcase. I gave her a quick rundown, mentioning again that my primary physician was setting up appointments for me with local specialists, but I wondered whether she had any other suggestions.

"I agree that you should start here," Susan said. "But it wouldn't hurt to get a second opinion in Boston."

Pikor had been at Amherst for more than a decade, and had forged close relationships with many trustees over the years. She told me that she was willing to check in with Dr. Frank Austen, a former trustee who was an emeritus professor of medicine at Harvard and who had chaired the department of rheumatology and immunology at the highly regarded Brigham and Women's Hospital in Boston.

Over the years, Dr. Austen had quietly provided referrals and made calls on behalf of people like myself who suddenly found themselves facing serious medical situations. "He's got a very good track record," Susan reassured me. "People he has helped over the years are doing quite well."

Her kindness floored me, and I thanked her for her assistance and her understanding. I was now ready to head home. My mind was racing, and I felt too agitated to concentrate on work. Despite it being a beautiful Friday afternoon, instead of the elation of heading off into the weekend after a productive week I felt like I was hurtling off into the unknown, leaving my comfortable routine behind for a future that was sure to include pain, suffering, and who knew what else.

• • •

A hypothetical: What exactly does one think about on the drive home when they've been diagnosed with what looks to be Stage IV cancer, the most serious and deadly of them all?

I've never asked anyone else that question. For my part, I thought about Katharina, and my two sons, Max and Jakob, and how much I loved my family.

Although I'm far from being a delusional optimist, I *do* try to find silver linings in bad situations. For me, a standard response to personal adversity is always, "It could be worse." And indeed, I thought about how fortunate I was that I had seen both of my sons grow up to be young men, had been very involved in raising them, and that my marriage to Katharina twenty-five years ago, when we were both so young, had endured and been strengthened over the years.

My mind also touched upon a number of other topics that would come to consume my attention in the coming weeks and months: *Would I be able to keep working? How was my health insurance? If illness forced me to quit working, did I have enough disability insurance through work and Social Security to pay the bills? Would it be difficult to get approved for a disability? How bad would my quality of life be? Would I ever be able to ski, run, swim, kayak, hike, run, or sail again? How will I tell Max and Jakob? How much information should I share with them?* The list of things to do seemed as endless as it was overwhelming.

As I dwelt on the financial side of things, the thought occurred to me that should the worst come to pass, at least my family would be taken care of. As it happened, my son Max worked as a financial adviser with Northwestern Mutual, where a big part of his job was explaining the benefits of life insurance to potential clients. And, about a month prior to all of this, he had persuaded me to buy a life insurance policy.

Admittedly, it didn't take much convincing. I was already proud of Max for taking on one of the toughest jobs there is—selling on pure commission—and I wanted to do my best to help him launch a successful career (and keep him from circling back to the nest as a twenty-something, if at all possible). I had been a life insurance skeptic for much of my adult life, but this was different: this was my own son making the case, and he had learned his lessons well.

Another silver lining. At least I have decent life insurance if I do die from this. Katharina and the boys will be taken care of.

• • •

As I pulled into the driveway of our house in Keene, I felt like I was entering a sanctuary. The property, which included a yard full of pear and apple trees, was perched on the edge of a ravine that led down to the West Branch of the Ashuelot River.

The house itself was simple yet solid, built shortly after World War II by an Italian immigrant who knew what he was doing. I felt comfortable here, as did the whole family. The old plan had been to put the house on the market in the spring and move to Amherst over the summer once Jakob had graduated from high school. A new chapter would then commence for Katharina and me, empty nesters in our mid-forties, embarking on an exciting new adventure in the more cosmopolitan environs of Amherst, Northampton and the other charming towns of the Pioneer Valley region. Now, I realized, those plans would have to be put on hold. There was no sense in moving if my very survival into the next year was in question.

Before I exited my car, I noticed that my Blackberry was blinking red, signaling an email. Hoping that it might be from Susan, perhaps with word from Dr. Frank Austen, I opened the message to read the words that would change the course of my treatment, and, I realize today, my life.

Peter,

Dr. Frank said that he will be glad to help. He asks that once you meet with the urologist and orthopedic surgeon, and based on your appointment with your primary care physician, to let us know the diagnosis your primary has in mind (as specifically as you can). Subsequently, Frank will consider your best options and be in touch with specialists with whom you might consult.

Call me when you can on Monday after your appointments.

Susan

This was good news—great news, even—and it made me hopeful. It also made me appreciate once more my boss and the college where I worked. The job wasn't perfect—what job is?—but what I held in my hands was nothing less than a powerful expression of support.

Collecting myself and my thoughts, I entered the house through the back and opened the back door to the kitchen. "Hello!" I called.

Katharina was in the dining room, but she came into the kitchen. I hugged her with my right arm, my left arm being too sore to lift. She squeezed me tight, and when I looked into her brown eyes, I saw my own fear and sadness mirrored.

Jakob came into the kitchen, and I hugged him tightly, too.

"Sorry to hear about this, dad," he said, his dark brown eyes, his mother's eyes, brimming with tears.

We all sat down at our round wood dining room table and looked at each other. In spite of it all, their fear gave me a kind of strength, reminding me that I needed to be strong for them, if not for myself.

"I'm going to fight this as hard as I can," I announced. "We'll get through this together, one day at a time."

Not particularly inspiring, I know. But even though I've made my living writing, working first as a journalist and later as an account executive/publicist, I've never been big on writing about myself or the challenges I've faced. My mandate is, and has always been, to present a cool façade to the outside world, remaining level-headed if at all possible.

What this meant was I didn't feel comfortable calling and telling people about my illness. All the same, I wanted those people who were or who had been close to me to know about it, because I wanted to believe that their good thoughts—and prayers, if they were religious—might help me heal. That perhaps, just maybe, their well wishes would send a message out into the universe that my spirit was worth tending to.

I also felt a deep sense of responsibility to my co-workers, and so before I went to bed that night, I sat down and wrote an email to my staff that was a variation of the language I would use for the next few days to spread the word about my illness.

And spread the word I did. The next morning, I emailed several of my colleagues at the college; I called my parents in Illinois, who still lived in the same house that I had grown up in about sixty miles west of Chicago; I sent emails to a few of my closest friends; I even called my aunt Kath, who lived nearby in Keene. Everyone got the same version of the story: Stage IV kidney cancer, major surgeries probable, followed by radiation, uncertain prognosis, details of exactly when my surgeries would occur still to be determined, doing my best to remain strong and positive, etc.

Of course, this isn't the sort of news a son *wants* to tell his aging parents or that an employee *wants* to share with his boss or colleagues. And although it was nourishing to hear their expressions of support, it was also draining for both Katharina and me.

At one point, after Katharina had made calls to her mother and two of her sisters in Austria, I found her crying.

"I'm scared about might happen," she confessed. "I feel like I was so naive in my life, thinking that I should be an artist."

It was then that I realized just how much she was worrying about how she would get by if I was unable to provide for her financially. Katharina worked as an adjunct professor at Keene State College, teaching drawing, design, and occasionally ceramics. Our home was filled with her beautiful ceramic dishware and sculptures; the lawn was festooned with ornaments, bird feeders, and sculptures, all made by her over the years. Drawings and paintings by her and our artist friends were framed and hung on our walls.

"I fell in love with you as an artist," I said, hugging her close. "You bring beauty and humanity into the world. There are more than enough accountants, lawyers, and businesspeople already. There aren't enough artists like you."

"You need to tell me that more often," she said, hugging me back. "And you need to write that down so that I can remember it if you're gone."

Later that day, my aunt Kath came by to pick up some orchids that Katharina had been tending while she and her husband Doug were in Florida. She also came to give me a hug.

"I'm so sorry," she said, her eyes welling with tears. It was getting to be quite a weepy time. "I feel I know you so well that it's like one of my own children giving me the news."

In the evening, my oldest son Max called from Burlington, Vermont, and we put him on speakerphone as Jakob, Katharina, and I sat down to dinner.

"How arc things, Max?" I asked.

"Not that good, really," Max replied. "My hand hurts."

"Why does your hand hurt?"

"I drank too much last night and I punched a wall."

"Why did you punch a wall?" Katharina asked.

"I was upset about things."

"What were you upset about?"

"I was upset about Dad."

Six years younger than his older brother and deeply sensitive, Jakob's voice was calm and firm as he laid out his perspective on my troubling diagnosis.

"One thing I'm focusing on is how much Dad has tried to help us, and is still trying to help us," he said. "Time is precious. Maybe we can think about how to make the most of it."

I added my bit: "Max, I can understand that you're mad. I'm mad myself. I'm mad that I was in good shape, that I've been working out and taking care of myself, and I've still got a tumor in my kidney, one on my arm, and one on my leg. I'm pissed about that."

I looked at Katharina and Jakob before continuing. "I'm mad that all of you have to go through this, because I know that while this disease affects me directly, it's also affecting you. My hope is that we can be strong together, supporting each other—and me, too. We all need to be strong."

"Hey, dad?" Max asked.

"Yeah?"

"I'm going to be mad about this for a while; I can't help that. But I'll be there for you, too. I know that we can fight this together."

"That sounds good, Max. One day at a time, right?"

We hung up and finished our dinner. On Monday, my medical journey would begin in earnest. But for the rest of the weekend, I'd focus on getting some rest and trying not to get too worried about the road ahead.

4 Local Docs

Over the weekend, I'd decided to approach my situation like the reporter I had once been. I would be a patient, but I would also ask questions and take notes. With that in mind, I made sure to bring along a digital tape recorder and a notebook to each of my appointments. *Who knows?* I thought. *If I come out okay on the other side, maybe I'll write a book about this someday.*

And so it was that Monday morning after Jakob headed off to school (and we'd brewed ourselves some much-needed coffee), Katharina and I set off to begin what we were calling "Day One" of my medical appointments. I hoped the day would yield more answers about my situation, my prognosis, and the treatment that lay ahead.

And maybe even some hope.

It had been exactly one week since my ill-fated slide on the ice (which had somehow led to a diagnosis of Stage IV cancer), and the weather had since warmed considerably. Rain pounded the windshield and combined with the melting snow to create a dense fog. The fifty-mile drive to our first appointment in Hatfield was like driving through a cloud bank. In fact, it was so foggy that I missed our exit and we were a few minutes late for my 9:30 am appointment with Dr. Jonathan Fallon, the orthopedic surgeon.

It didn't really matter, as it turned out. The waiting room was already full of patients, many with arms in casts, feet in plastic support boots, and crutches at their sides. Compared to them, I looked fine. Broken bones could be set, after all. Tendons could be sewed or stapled back together. I was reminded of my own orthopedic repairs over the years, which included ruptures of my Achilles tendons, five years apart, while playing basketball.

Meanwhile, my cancer had already eaten away at one bone and was beginning to do the same to another. And who knew where it would show up next?

I wish all I had was a broken leg or a ruptured Achilles tendon. Those were the days.

Despite my gloomy mood, I had actually gained some perspective on my situation. Over the weekend, Katharina and I had had occasion to count our blessings, and we realized that while I did have cancer, I was also fortunate enough to have access to cancer treatment options that many others didn't. Amherst College, my employer, not only provided excellent health insurance, but because of its location in Massachusetts, offered access to some of the best cancer treatment in the world. As a result, I had the option to pursue a second opinion at Dana-Farber and maybe even get treated there. The plastic Blue Cross/Blue Shield card in my wallet was a talisman that would grant me access to world-class treatment.

After about fifteen minutes, my name was called, and a nurse's aide led Katharina and me into an examining room to wait for Dr. Fallon.

He walked into the examining room a short time later, wearing the white lab coat that seemed to be the official uniform of all physicians, though I could remember reading studies that found lab coats and neck ties to be mobile breeding grounds for all sorts of nasty germs. I tried to put that out of my mind as Dr. Fallon greeted us warmly with a confident hello and a hearty handshake.

"Thanks for coming in," he said after we'd exchanged introductions. "I haven't seen the whole report, but I have seen the scans. It showed me enough, especially the bone scans. It looks like you have a little something lighting up above your knee and a big goober in your humerus."

Interesting terminology, I thought. "So when you say 'big goober,' what do you mean exactly?"

"A big lesion, right here," he said, pointed to an image of my scan. "You can see how the bone looks normal here, and this looks kind of irregular down here?" he asked. "But if you look at the images from the bone scan, it's much more telling. That's the lesion up in the arm," he said, gesturing to an area of the scan. "That's the painful one.

"Now this is the one right above the right knee," he continued, moving on. "Do you feel anything from that?"

"Not really," I said. "But what about the arm—can you tell how vulnerable that is to fracture? The radiologist seemed pretty freaked about that in his report."

The images were no less alarming, showing two darkened areas where the radioactive tracer that had been injected into me before the scan had accumulated in greater amounts, indicating cancerous lesions.

"Well, radiologists are radiologists," Dr. Fallon said dismissively, not bothering to elaborate, but hinting at what I would come to learn was a stereotypical description: that radiologists spent their days in small, dark rooms examining image after image, detached from the patients that they represented. In other words, radiologists were the "antisocial geeks" of the M.D. world.

And if that was the case, then orthopedic surgeons were the extroverted jocks—at least, if Dr. Fallon was any indication.

Returning to my original question, Dr. Fallon pointed at the bone scan image again. "See, here? This is normal bone cortex, which you lose...*there*. Which is most definitely something to give pause. I don't see a definitive fracture, but this is absolutely at risk for pathological fracture."

"And a fracture would open a whole new can of worms?" I hazarded.

"Yes and no," he replied. "It's more of a pain issue. The affected part of the bone is not solid and the bone itself is flexible, and that's not good for bone. Quite painful, in fact.

"Normally, if this were to break, we'd put you in a sling and you'd heal. The problem is that you're not going to heal through a tumor. So what we would typically do is treat the tumor through radiation—so long as you had no symptoms—and the bone would remodel. But since your arm *isn't* functional, there's reason to do the surgery."

Now we were getting to the question that every website I'd visited told me to ask: how many surgeries had the surgeon done?

(Of course, this is a chicken and egg scenario. How is a surgeon supposed to get experience if no one wants a novice for a surgeon? But that wasn't my problem; I wanted an experienced surgeon to be the one driving a titanium nail through the center of my cancerous humerus bone.)

"Is this a type of surgery you have experience doing?" I asked.

"Yes," he replied with a confident smile.

"And how many of them have you done?"

"Humeral nails? I've done a total of four in my life," he said. "Three of them for pathological fractures like yours and one for just a fracture. It's not an overly complicated surgery; the hard part is realigning the bone, and your bone is already aligned."

"What about the interaction with the tumor? I've heard there are orthopedic surgeons who specialize in oncology."

Dr. Fallon leaned back in his chair. "So here's the question I would want to pose: does this need to be biopsied? Is the tumor in your arm the source tumor, or is it a metastatic lesion? Based on the CT scan, it *looks* like a metastatic lesion, and if that's the case I'm comfortable taking care of it.

"However, if there's a possibility that this *is* a primary tumor, then an orthopedic oncologist would need to be involved. I happen to know an excellent orthopedic oncologist at U-Mass Medical Center in Worcester—Dr. Matthew Most. I could easily get you into see him, or we could even start off with him, and that's fine, too. My job is to get you as comfortable as possible and let the hematologist-oncologist deal with the cancer. If you're more comfortable seeing an orthopedic oncologist, I have no problem with that. No need to worry about my ego," he added with a smile.

Katharina and I exchanged looks. We both knew that seeing specialists in Boston was still on the table, and as soon as we heard he'd performed this surgery less than half a dozen times, we were on the same wavelength. Dr. Fallon was a nice guy, sure, and his confidence was appreciated, but it didn't look like he'd be the one performing *my* surgery.

What that meant was it was time to ask whatever questions we had while making sure we didn't commit to anything. Our planned trip to Belize was still in the works, after all. Katharina had spent hours planning that trip; neither of us wanted to give up on it just yet.

"My question is about what he can do until he gets the surgery," Katharina said. "Two people have already warned us it's so fragile that it could break, and we're very active people. Is there a support he can wear to protect his arm? What can he reasonably do to protect himself?"

"Well," Dr. Fallon said, looking out the window, "not that it's an issue given the rain, but cross-country skiing, for example, is a bad idea. But getting on a bicycle is reasonable, assuming you don't fall off."

"We actually have a trip coming up for our twenty-fifth wedding anniversary, to Belize. We were hoping to do some kayaking and swimming."

"Swimming and light snorkeling is okay," he said after a moment's thought. "I would not get on a kayak; you wouldn't want to flip. But overall? At this point, I would say go and enjoy yourselves; I certainly can't fix this before you go. But I would stay away from anything where you'd have to rely on that arm for support."

"Good thing we cut bungee jumping out of the itinerary," Katharina joked. "Maybe we'll just sit on the beach with a tropical drink or a glass of wine."

"Wine's also a good blood thinner to prevent clots on the plane," Dr. Fallon said with a smile as he prepared to make his leave. "I highly recommend a good red."

"Thanks for being so encouraging about our trip," I said as we stood to leave. "Dr. Wu and the radiologist both said we shouldn't go."

"Well, there's your first problem right there. Don't talk to a radiologist," Dr. Fallon advised, and stuck his hand out for a farewell shake. "They don't see patients, they see x-rays."

•   •   •

After that largely positive encounter, our next appointment was in Florence, a small town embedded into Northampton. We were headed to see Dr. Donald Sonn, the urologist who would be removing my right kidney if I chose to remain local with my care. After spending the weekend reading about the grim prognosis for Stage IV kidney cancer patients, we were nervously anticipating this appointment.

Dr. Sonn had been recommended by Dr. Wu as being compassionate and highly qualified to perform what was likely to be a necessary nephrectomy. The Chief Surgeon at Cooley Dickinson Hospital, Dr. Sonn's profile noted his expertise in treating impotence, removing kidney stones, and using robotic surgery to treat prostate cancer. We arrived after lunch to find the waiting room empty and were quickly led into an examining room, a setting already all too familiar.

"The first thing you need to do," Dr. Sonn began, after listening to my diagnosis, "is think about getting plugged into an oncologist."

I told him that my boss had been tapping into her network to see whether she could get me a referral at Dana-Farber or somewhere else in Boston. I felt he should know that I was considering all options, including the importance of receiving coordinated care, especially given the complicated nature of the two surgeries I was facing.

He reassured me, as Dr. Fallon had, that there was no need to concern myself with his ego. "I want you to get the best care possible," he said, "regardless of whether it's here or elsewhere. We send a lot of patients to Dana-Farber; they have a world-class oncology program. I tell all my patients to get second opinions, even third opinions. There really should be no limit to the amount of discussion about this."

"On the other hand," I replied, thinking of the tumors growing in various places in my body, "we *are* racing the clock a bit, aren't we?"

"I'm not sure if we're racing the clock, but we do want to expedite things," he said. "I'm not sure the specialists at Dana-Farber are going to tell you anything different. That said, the advantage of the really large institutions is they can plug you into clinical trials. The problem with clinical trials, however, is it's sort of like coin toss as to whether you'll get a placebo."

The notion sounded horrifying. A 50-50 chance I'd be getting a sugar pill?

"They wouldn't do that with cancer, would they?" Katharina asked.

"It's possible," he said. "Or else, they might put you in some experimental therapy that doesn't have any proven results.

"The other advantage with going to Dana-Farber, though, is that you gain more information about all of this. While I'd be very surprised if they told you they had a new treatment that's much different than what has already been suggested, I still think it would be very helpful to go to there, if only because kidney cancer is such a weird type of cancer. In a small number of cases, people do really well. In some patients it even spontaneously regresses."

Dr. Sonn adjusted his glasses before asking, "How old are you?"

"Forty-six," I answered.

"I had this one young guy about ten years ago; he was actually twenty-nine at the time he was diagnosed. Very similar case to yours. The cancer had spread to his bones, and when we took out his kidney, we found it was a real large tumor. About twice as large as yours. He was put on tyrosine kinase inhibitors and he's still alive today. But while we have those types of responses, we also have other people who *don't* have good responses. It's important to keep that in mind."

"So you've seen people come back from this?" I asked. I was still looking to find some hope in all this.

Dr. Sonn nodded. "Even though the prognosis is very tough and very guarded, with these new treatments, I'm more optimistic."

"And one more thing," he added. "I wouldn't look at the Internet for any of this information. It's all outdated, not to mention it's kind of depressing to be looking at the old five-year survival rates."

"It's less than ten percent on the Internet," Katharina said.

"I would say it's higher than that. If you respond well to some of the tyrosine-kinase inhibitor drugs, you have a decent shot at this."

Finally, we broached the 'Belize question.' "There's a trip we've been planning to celebrate our twenty-fifth wedding anniversary," I said. "We were going to leave on Saturday for a week in Belize. Is that really stupid and irresponsible?"

"No," said Dr. Sonn, "I don't think so at all. I'm just a little worried that you won't be able to move your arm."

"Well, I'd protect it," I said. "I'm not planning to do any scuba diving or kayaking. I was thinking I'd try to line up as many medical appointments as I can beforehand and then enjoy a week on the beach before dealing with all of this."

Dr. Sonn's final words on the subject were encouraging yet grim. "You should enjoy your vacation," he said as he saw us off. "This has been brewing for a long time. A week is not going to change things that much."

5 A Call from Boston

The oncologist from the Dana-Farber Cancer Center was equally optimistic regarding our trip to the tropics.

He introduced himself over the phone as Dr. Toni Choueiri, his voice sounding confident and welcoming with a hint of a central European accent (which turned out to be Lebanese). He was calling at the suggestion of a retired physician and former Amherst College trustee who my boss had approached for a referral.

I felt a deep and instant gratitude for this doctor, who was taking time out on a late afternoon to call and offer to take me on as his patient. All the more so, as I was still debating whether or not to stay local with my treatment or else drive the ninety miles or so into Boston to go to Dana-Farber (or even work out some sort of hybrid model, where some of the treatment took place locally and the rest occurred in Boston).

"Local," of course, would not be in Keene, New Hampshire, but would take place at Cooley Dickinson Hospital in Northampton, Massachusetts, about an hour's drive to the south. Because my health insurance coverage was only valid in Massachusetts, I would be driving a considerable distance for my care no matter what option I chose.

"I would recommend that you come here," Dr. Choueiri said. "If you say no, that's fine—I'm in tune with the medical

31

community there and I can work with them. But personally, I don't have any privileges at Cooley Dickinson. So my suggestion would be to come here for treatment."

He paused, before getting to the heart of the matter. "They tell me you have a kidney mass and that it has spread to the bone, correct?"

"That's what the initial CT scan shows, yes," I replied.

"In one place?"

"Two places, unfortunately. I have a smaller lesion in my right femur."

"I see," he said, and considered for a moment. "I think you need a firm course of action for your care, and I don't think you should be jumping from one place to another. That's not a good thing. Going back and forth between doctors just complicates things.

"And speaking of complications, I understand more you're going on a trip, right?"

"We had planned a trip, yes," I said. "We were going to be leaving this Saturday. It's only for a week, but if you don't think it's a good idea..."

"In all honesty, Peter, I think it's okay," he reassured me. "I don't think anything bad will happen in a week. At least as far as your kidneys go. As for your arm...I don't have access to those pictures yet, but you know that if you break it there, that's a big headache.

"But it's up to you. If it's such an important trip that if you feel you need to go, a week will not make a big difference. That said if something *does* happen there in Belize...well, I'd be surprised if they have an oncologist there.

"I think the first thing you need to do," he continued, moving on to matters more in line with his specialty, "is to have those bones addressed. You'll need the standard battery of tests, followed by the kidney itself being removed, followed by seeing me. I work with a lot of specialists that can do all of this."

"So the bones to be addressed—that would be in the Boston area?" I asked.

"That's right, because the Brigham and Dana-Farber are one."

"So that would be a surgery by someone with experience working around a tumor in the bone, right?"

"*Of course,*" he replied, in a tone that suggested the very question was borderline offensive. "This is the Brigham and Women's Hospital. We're a tertiary care hospital that has fifteen orthopedic surgeons who specialize in cancer. People come from all over the world, not just from Boston, to receive treatment."

This all sounded great to me, and we made the appointment then and there for the Tuesday after we got back from Belize. He also told me to anticipate a call from their patient coordinator, a woman named Jean Kirwan, who would start pulling my records and putting together a file on my case.

Finally, he asked, "Have you had a biopsy performed?"

"No, I haven't."

"Okay. That's something that *can* be done at Cooley Dickinson," he said. "In fact, if they can do a biopsy this week, that would be great. That way, by the time you get back we will have an idea of what's going on.

"I can tell you that in ninety percent of cases, cancer of the kidney is going to present as what's called 'clear cell renal cell carcinoma.' But, as in a small percentage of cases, this may end up being a strange cancer of the kidney which will require different treatment."

"Is the biopsy a surgery, then?"

"No," he replied, "it's all outpatient. It's very simple."

I told him I'd do my best to get an appointment in place before we left for Belize, already relieved by the way that Dr. Choueiri had calmly taken charge of the situation and put a plan for treatment in place.

I thanked him for his time and for the leadership role he'd assumed in my care. "No worries," he said. "We'll take care of you. But do understand—this is not something to take lightly. I *do* think we will be able to help you better here. This is nothing against the place you are at now, but sometimes we can help patients more when we have more expertise."

"That sounds good to me," I said.

• • •

Just two days later, Dr. George Hartnell, an interventional radiologist at Cooley Dickinson, was inserting a long, hollow needle into my right kidney. By doing so, he was able to extract a core sample of my tumor for analysis, so my cancer could be assessed and categorized.

I was lying on my belly, having been carefully arranged into position on the gurney before getting pushed beneath the whirring donut shape of the Siemens CT scanning machine.

Before we began, he asked whether we had any questions.

"Can you promise a miraculous recovery?" Katharina asked, which was putting him somewhat on the spot, I thought. Still, I was curious to hear his answer.

"I don't promise miracles," he said, a bit dour. "However, if there ever was hope for a miraculous recovery, it would be with kidney cancer tumors. I've seen them clear up very nicely."

Katharina and I both liked that answer, and I gave her hand a squeeze before heading into the donut hole.

What I liked far less was the pain in my right flank that I felt when the local anesthesia wore off. It was more intense than I had anticipated, and I knew it was only a hint of the pain that was likely to come.

I didn't go to work the next day, instead downing a Vicodin every few hours as I tried to look at the positives. For one thing, the day off gave me time more time to pack. As I did so, I began looking forward to leaving the grey New England winter behind for a sunny resort in Belize. Soon we would be enjoying the beaches, ensconced in a thatch roof hut right on the water. I was determined: no sore kidney or slightly fractured arm was going to stop me from relaxing for a week to get myself prepared for the grueling surgeries and treatment ahead.

Or so I thought.

6 Visiting Dana-Farber

I t's probably for the best that the trip to Belize didn't happen, but at the time it was quite devastating, especially for Katharina, who had spent hours researching possibilities and making the arrangements online. But in an era of being your own travel agent, pulling off a trip without some sort of glitch in the logistics requires a minor miracle.

"Katharina," I called from our bedroom, where I was stuffing shorts, t-shirts, and a pair of flip-flops into a rolling suitcase, "I think we should go ahead and print our boarding passes."

I zipped up my suitcase and carefully carried it downstairs, my left arm dangling limply at my side. I heard the printer whirring and set the suitcase down before retrieving the freshly printed boarding passes. I glanced them over, looking to confirm that the printout was clean and legible, when I noticed something odd. While there *were* boarding passes for each of us from Hartford to Philadelphia, there was only one from Philadelphia to Belize City.

I carried the pages into the dining room, where Katharina was sitting at the laptop.

"Can you check the itinerary and make sure both of us are booked for Belize and back?" I asked. "There's only one boarding pass, for you."

"Just a second," she said. A few keyboard clicks later she said, "Oh, no."

"That doesn't sound good."

"It isn't," she said. "I don't see your name on the itinerary for the flight to Belize. That's...very strange. I know that I *paid* for tickets for both of us."

"I'm sure you booked tickets for both of us, too," I said. "Do you want to call Expedia, or should I?"

Katharina and I are effective at what we do, but neither of us are great negotiators. We'd rather not deal with the give-and-take of sealing a deal if we can help it. Not to mention that neither one of us was at our best right now. After a week of medical appointments, with a diagnosis of Stage IV kidney cancer still sinking in, we just wanted to get on a plane to someplace warm.

From the beginning, the exchange with Expedia was a circular conversation. I argued that we had both purchased tickets to Belize and back, while the customer service rep at the other end, in the detached, slightly bored voice that seems to be part of their job description, assured me that that no, we hadn't.

She repeatedly added, as I questioned her politely at first but with then with growing anger, frustration, and ultimately resignation, that the only way for me to make the trip to Belize was to buy a ticket for a different flight at an additional cost of $2,100, as the flight I *wanted* to be on was full.

In a dazed and slightly befuddled state, Katharina and I considered our options. Katharina's eyes were red from silent crying as she heard me trying, to no avail, to salvage something from our predicament.

I think we reached a similar conclusion at about the same time—it just wasn't meant to be. If it meant eating the cost of our trip, then so be it. The karma for this trip sucked, and so we decided to pull the plug on it.

Before, I had been worrying about how my left arm and shoulder would weather the strain of hoisting my carry-on bag into the overhead compartment. Now, I thought with guilty relief, at least my shoulder won't be subjected to more jostling. And I would be able to work on scheduling my medical appointments earlier. *What joy.*

As I lay in bed that night, waiting for sleep to come, my thoughts turned reluctantly from the sunny beaches and coral reefs of Belize to the still raw March of New England and the doctors in Boston who—I hoped—held the key to my survival.

•   •   •

My ability to salvage our trip to Belize notwithstanding, I've always been pretty good at working around obstacles, making the best of the situation at hand no matter how demoralizing it may seem.

That said, I'm not delusional either. If the writing's on the wall, Not to mix metaphors, but I'm willing to throw in the towel. What was making my current situation difficult was determining how *much* hope was realistic. The Internet didn't provide much help, and neither did the extra time I suddenly found myself with, now that I wasn't relaxing on the beach.

I knew I needed to get moving on my treatment, and so I decided I would try to turn my thwarted trip into an opportunity to get a jump-start on that process. The way I saw it, the sooner my cancerous kidney could be removed and my arm repaired—preferably in one hospital stay which would be horrendous but would at least it would be over relatively quickly—the sooner could I focus on getting better and doing my best to kick cancer's ass.

First thing Monday morning, I called Jean Kirwan, the patient coordinator at Dana-Farber. I was expecting I'd need to fill her in on my situation, but it turned out Dr. Choueiri had already taken care of that.

In fact, Kirwan had already begun scheduling appointments for me three weeks out, but she seamlessly switched gears when I told her that the next two weeks were now suddenly open for me. Three days later, Katharina and I were seated in a brand-spanking-new examining room on the twelfth floor of Dana-Farber's gleaming Yawkey Center for Cancer Care. It even smelled new, the $330 million glass and terra cotta-clad building having only opened to patients a few weeks earlier.

Dr. Choueiri bounded into the room with a toothy smile, exuding confidence and energy. He wasted little time with formalities and plunged into a quick recap of my situation in his slightly accented English. His manner was straightforward and compassionate, which I appreciated. Also, he had researched and published on kidney cancer extensively, and I appreciated that even more. Despite his relatively youthful appearance, Dr. Choueiri was already a leading kidney cancer researcher and clinician.

"What this seems to be," he said, zeroing in on the matter after we had made our introductions, "is a kidney cancer. Kidney cancer comes in multiple flavors; this is the most common type, renal clear cell cancer. What's more, we're sure that this has spread outside the kidney. Based on what we saw while evaluating the scans, it seems to be in two spots so far—one in your left humerus, and one in your right leg. Right leg, left arm, in other words."

Dr. Choueiri paused and I nodded. He continued, explaining that the first step in my treatment would be fixing my left arm. "That procedure will be performed by Dr. Marco Ferrone, and will happen soon," he said. "After that, the kidney needs to come out, which will be done by Dr. Steven Chang." He concluded his recap by saying, "There *is* a possibility that both operations would happen at the same time or close to it."

"That's what we're hoping," Katharina said.

"There are some technical issues, though," he continued. "They can't put you in the air to take your kidney. What I mean is they'll need to have you lying on your side during that procedure, which means you would be leaning on your left shoulder. How we choose to approach that issue will be decided by Dr. Ferrone and Dr. Chang talking together. We'll then have all the pathology, after which you'll have to come back and see me because we'll want to take a close look at the other leg."

Dr. Choueiri ran off a list of tests he wanted me to have done at Dana-Farber: a brain MRI to see whether I had any brain tumors (because kidney cancer is known to spread to the brain), another set of x-rays of my left arm and right leg, and a blood draw. He gave detailed instructions to his resident, Elizabeth Guancial, before turning back to us.

"What I want to tell you today is this: there are reasons to be worried and there are reasons to hope," he said. "It's possible that this is a cancer that cannot be cured, and that it has already spread. That's what a Stage IV diagnosis entails. But there *are* reasons to hope. It seems to be in only two places, and there is a chance—though I don't know how high it is—to take the kidney out and really work on those two lesions with radiation. There's a chance that, after that, nothing else needs to happen. And, even if we fail in that plan and the cancer spreads to other places, there are drugs we can give you that will potentially put this disease in remission. For how long, we don't know. It could be months or even years. So there *is* hope for a kidney cancer patient in this day and age."

"What about chemo?" I asked him.

"This is different than other cancers," he replied. "Chemo is not a treatment we use in kidney cancer; it doesn't work."

The reason for this, as I found out later, is because kidney cancer cells are very porous, which means the chemotherapy can't build up in high enough levels to be toxic to tumors. On the plus side, this characteristic also makes kidney cancer cells more vulnerable to targeted therapies that block off the blood supply to tumors. That said, while these treatments can work for a year or two, the cancer cells inevitably evolve to the point where they can develop new pathways to obtain the blood that nourishes their growth and ensures their survival.

I mulled over everything he told me before saying, "I have Stage IV cancer and I want to be as positive as possible, while staying realistic. What do I have going for me?"

"What you have going for you is that you're in good health and the cancer didn't spread to many places. Working against you is the fact that renal cell cancer, when it does spread, is not curable. We can potentially extend your life, but it is hard to know for sure, or for how long. This is an area where research is still being done, and there are always new drugs being produced that can get patients into another remission, for a time."

The situation was once again sinking in.

"So at this point, it's not curable?" Katharina asked.

"Most likely, no," the doctor replied. "But there is a chance that we can address each of these issues individually and perhaps cure it. It's a not a big possibility—it's a small possibility, in fact--but it exists."

"What if we do nothing?" Katharina asked.

"I wouldn't advise that. I'd put your prognosis at less than a year, without treatment. With treatment, there's a potential for extended life.

"I will be very honest with you at every step of your treatment. If you ask me, 'Will I be around in five years?' the answer is it's hard to know. If this had happened ten years ago, probably not. But now we have a lot more options."

Katharina looked at me with tears in her eyes, and Dr. Choueiri offered her a tissue.

"Hang in there," he said, addressing me as well. "This is *not* a death sentence. It's something that came out of nowhere and it's unfair, no doubt about that. My suggestion is to take things day by day. If you want to work and you have a desk job, continue doing it, but know that you'll be taking days and even weeks off, taking care of the kidney and the arm. Remember that things can change every time—you can have something new." He smiled. "One drug could give you six months to a year, another could give you twelve months, and after those two years we could have found a miracle cure. That's the beauty of receiving treatment at a research institution. Think about it like that."

"That does sound good," I admitted. "I believe in positive thinking, as long as it's not delusional thinking." I stopped and added, my tone carefully neutral, "What do you think about that, by the way? How important is positive thinking or a good attitude?"

"The power of positive thinking can definitely help with cancer," he said. "We have the data to support that. Know also that you are not alone; there are people at Dana-Farber and at Brigham who can help you. We have an extensive network of support groups and social workers, all specializing in this disease. A lot of my patients have been alive for many years, and they can help you, too."

Seeing that he had settled us down, at least on the surface, he stood to leave. "And maybe next year you can try for Belize again! This time, take me with you, okay? I've never been."

"Me, neither, "I said, "But maybe next year."

It wouldn't be easy. I knew that, and so did Katharina. But if an oncologist at Dana-Farber said there was hope, then Katharina and I were going to take him at his word.

7 Surgical Planning

Afer that it was off to Dr. Steven Chang for a consultation about my cancerous kidney. Dr. Chang had earned his medical degree from Columbia University and been a resident at Stanford, all of which served to reassure me I'd be receiving a quality of care in line with what Dana-Farber promised.

"I took a look at the notes on your case," he said, gesturing to a computer monitor displaying my latest CT scan results. "You were in your normal state of health until you started feeling some pain. Is that right?"

"That's right, "I said. "I was pretty active—skiing, downhill and cross-country skiing, working out at the gym, swimming laps. I started feeling shoulder pain whenever I did the freestyle over-hand stroke and when I did pull-ups, to the point where I went to my primary care doctor and asked for a physical therapy referral. I just thought it was sore."

"And this was in late February?"

I shook my head. "This would have been late January. I started working with the PT, and he gave me some range of motion exercises that seemed to be helping.

"Then, on February 28, the Monday after a skiing trip, I was driving into work and I hit a patch of ice. I jerked the steering wheel with my left hand and there was a shot of searing pain right around here." I pointed to my upper arm. "That's what got this ball rolling."

I looked closely at the youthful Dr. Chang. "Listen, before we go any further," I said, trying to get a read on this person who would be extracting a vital organ from my body, "I have a question. I'm guessing you've seen quite a few people in my situation. What sort of outcome can I expect after all of the surgeries and treatments are over?"

"The best outcomes for patients in this type of situation are often determined by their underlying health, and it doesn't get much healthier than you," he replied. "Swimming, doing pull-ups— these are things that we would love to see every patient do. So I can virtually guarantee that you'll recover well from orthopedic surgery in addition to the type of surgery I'm talking about. You will recover from the systemic therapy well."

I like this guy, I thought. *Confident, though maybe a little cocky.*

"What about the long term picture?" I asked.

"In terms of the long-term outlook, a lot of that is based on the biology of the disease and how it's spread. Our goal is to cure you of this disease, and our expectation is that you're going to have a long, happy life. The first step is to get rid of the primary tumor area, which means taking out the kidney." He paused. "Well, actually, our first step is to take care of the orthopedic issues, but getting rid of this primary tumor is the first phase of your recovery. After which Dr. Choueiri's expertise in terms of systemic therapy will start to play a major role."

This was exactly what I was looking for—evidence of collaboration and coordinated communication. I could sense that my problems crossed several medical specialties, and appreciated the benefits of complementary care.

"The beauty of being here at the Dana-Farber," Dr. Chang continued, "is that there's no pressure to move on to the next patient until we're completely done. I work with people in different fields, including the medical oncologists and radiation oncologists. And while we all have different ways of treating things, everything's very equitable. Everyone just puts their opinion out, and there's no struggle over territory."

Sure, it was a bit of a sales pitch, but it turned out to be true— not only was communication strong among the Dana-Farber folks, when the time came later to hand me off to an immune therapy specialist at another cancer clinic in Boston, there was no hesitation. I found out later that many of those who specialize in kidney cancer consider themselves to be collaborators and often work together on research funded by the National Cancer Institute.

Dr. Chang made it clear that his job would pretty much be confined to the nephrectomy, the removal of my kidney, which he viewed as the best way to deal with the primary tumor.

"I look at the kidney—where the tumor is, the size of it—and I try to determine whether I can remove just that part of the kidney, or if the whole kidney needs to go. This one in particular is really on the borderline. See here?" he asked, pointing to a specific spot on the scan, near the dark blotch that represented the tumor. "If I just remove that part, we run the risk of injuring the nearby blood vessels that feed the kidney. Damage those, and the rest of the kidney might end up deteriorating."

For that reason, Dr. Chang recommended taking out the entire kidney with a laparoscopic procedure, which would save me considerable healing pain.

"We perform the surgery through small, keyhole-shaped incisions," he explained. "We're following the same principles as the original so-called 'open procedure.' We transect the vessels that feed the kidney, and then we basically remove the whole thing, along with the surrounding fat. The major benefit of this procedure is the short recovery period; patients are typically released after two to three days, after they've reached three major milestones: eating solid foods, tolerating the pain well enough to be removed from a morphine IV drip, and being able to walk."

"This is not any kind of marathon walk, either," he told Katharina and me. "This is just feeling confident enough to get up and take a few steps. At that point, there's not much you're doing in the hospital that you couldn't do for yourself at home."

As far as the recovery itself, Dr. Chang said the first two weeks were the hardest, and that most patients felt pretty good after about four weeks. He also said there was no reason to believe that my left kidney, which looked perfectly healthy, wouldn't pick up the slack for its departed partner.

"I have every reason to believe that you can do very well with one kidney, but we'll still keep an eye on it, and not take anything for granted," he said. "In ten, fifteen, twenty years, I want to make sure that you're still doing well."

Talking about the long term, I thought. *I like that. Even if he does sound a bit delusional.*

•   •   •

Our next appointment was with Dr. Marco Ferrone, an orthopedic surgeon with an oncology specialty. He certainly looked the part; Dr. Ferrone was like a surgeon from central casting—the literal "Mr. Tall, Dark, and Handsome."

His voice was deep and authoritative, yet quiet; so quiet I had to lean in to hear him when he sat down with us in his examining room. He had an air of solemnity, which conveyed a sense of respect for the serious situations his patients encountered.

He began by asking me questions about my medical history and lifestyle habits. The usual questions: "Do you smoke?" *(Tried but never developed the habit for it)*; "Do you drink alcohol?" *(A couple drinks a day);* "Drink soda?" *(Not very often.)*

He then presented us with a matter-of-fact description of the operation. He'd begin by separating the tissues and tendons in my shoulder to gain access to the top center of my humerus so that he could guide a long titanium nail through to the elbow, after which he would stabilize everything with pins.

As an orthopedic surgeon with a specialty in bone metastases, it was an operation he had performed many times before, and he didn't anticipate any problems with this one. Better yet, Dr. Ferrone said he would be consulting with Dr. Chang and Dr. Choueiri, but in his opinion it was possible have my right kidney removed during the same hospital stay.

"I think we can position you so your left shoulder and arm will be protected," he said. "You seem to be in good health, and there's something to be said for getting this all over with so you can focus on healing and the radiation treatment that will follow."

Looking at my arm, which even now hung limply from my side, I asked, "How strong can I expect my arm to be? What sort of range of motion can I expect to get back?"

"In terms of strength, that really depends on how the bone heals around the nail," he answered. "If it heals well, it will be good for many years. Your range of notion might not be quite what it was, but gains there can vary widely."

"I'll also be getting radiation to my right knee; do you think there's a danger of a break there any time soon?"

Dr. Ferrone sat back in his chair. "It's going to do what it does," he replied. "I'm not going to say it will break no matter what, because it may never break. I also think exercise is a *good* thing. If you were to put yourself in a bubble with zero gravity, your bones would disintegrate. Bones *need* exercise; they need that stress and that loading to maintain themselves. I'm not saying you should go play sports, but walking, biking, things like that? Go for it. Though," he added, "I wouldn't do anything where you're likely to fall."

"No more skiing for a while then," I said and grinned faintly. "Oh, well. The season's almost over, anyway."

Looking back, it was this appointment that gave me the confidence and motivation to come back from my surgeries with a focus on exercise. In truth, I was already planning to be less cautious than what Dr. Ferrone was recommending. My goal was to return to my normal activities—which including skiing, swimming, and kayaking—as soon as possible after the radiation.

At least, that was the plan.

8 Under the Knife

I woke up in my own comfortable bed, ready to greet a clear Saturday morning, once more relieved that we had bailed on Belize. My left arm seemed more sore than ever, especially now that I could so clearly visualize how much of my humerus had been eaten away.

I'm very impressionable that way.

Even tamping fresh ground coffee and slotting the metal double-shot filter into the espresso machine brought intense pain to my bicep and shoulder. It was a sacrifice I was willing to make—nothing tastes better than the first morning coffee—but it did drive home for me again just how much my daily life was affected by my illness.

I sat down at our round dining room table and reviewed my situation. My fervent hope was that the titanium nail implant would help make my left arm reasonably functional and strong again. Following that, I would recover from my kidney surgery and the radiation to my arm and knee would kill whatever cancer was stirring there, all while allowing my bones to rejuvenate themselves.

It was a tall order, but to me it seemed like a reasonable thing to hope for—a path for my mind and body to follow. If all that happened, I reasoned, I could return to my active lifestyle, which would help build up my immune system. That, in turn, would keep my mind and body strong, allowing me to live long enough to hopefully see Jakob graduate from the University of Vermont, where he planned to enroll in the fall, joining his older brother in Burlington.

Four years. An eternity, really—especially considering my current medical situation. I couldn't help picturing myself bedridden and wondered whether I would be able to adapt and accept that situation.

You won't have a choice, I thought. *But that hasn't happened yet, so quit worrying about it.*

• • •

And in fact, there was some reason to be hopeful. I'd received the results of the pathology report from my recent biopsy, which grades kidney cancer for their aggressiveness. Mine had graded out as a 2, on a scale of 1 to 4. Not too bad.

I also had the most common type of kidney cancer, renal clear cell carcinoma, which accounted for about eighty percent of kidney cancer diagnoses. That meant that the bulk of the resources allocated to kidney cancer research and treatment were focused on my condition. Kidney cancer is considered to be a quirky disease, with wide variations in survival rates among those diagnosed. I was pinning my hopes on having a slow-growing cancer that I could fend off by boosting my immune system through regular exercise and good nutrition.

As for my mental health, I was working on that, too. My spirits were lifted by calls, emails, and cards from colleagues, family, and friends, but I remained scared about the future. The five-year survival rate for kidney cancer that I had encountered most often on the Internet was a cripplingly low ten percent.

When I had mentioned this figure to Dr. Choueiri during my appointment, he had been quick to dispute it.

"That figure is based on old data, and fails to take into account some of the more recent treatments," he told me. "And there's another thing you'll notice: the term median survival is used a lot. With cancer, there's a lot of luck involved. Median survival is how long a person with average luck will live, based on the data that's available.

"You were unlucky to get cancer, there's no question about that, but now that you are in our care, it's our job to figure out the best treatment for you. I know it's hard not to worry, but that is what I would recommend to you, if at all possible."

It *was* a tall order, but as the minutes, hours, and days slowly passed, I tried to keep my mind free of unnecessary worry (though I frequently caught myself wishing for better-than-average luck).

The phone rang as I savored my coffee. It was a receptionist from Dr. Ferrone's office, calling to tell me my surgery would take place that Thursday. A couple hours later, Dr. Chang called me from his cellphone to say he was scheduling my nephrectomy for Saturday afternoon, in exactly one week.

"That way you'll have a couple days to recover from your shoulder surgery," he said.

"Really?" I asked. "Coming in on a Saturday—you're sure you don't mind?"

"Did you hear about the face transplant operation we did last week?"

The operation, the nation's first full face transplant, had taken place the previous weekend at Brigham and Women's and had been a top medical story that week all over the country.

"If they could do a face transplant over the weekend, I can do a kidney removal," Dr. Chang said. "We all agree that it would be optimal to remove the kidney and fix your shoulder in the same hospital stay. That way, you'll heal more quickly and then proceed to radiation and other treatment more quickly, too. We wouldn't recommend this for everyone, but you're young and—except for the cancer—healthy. You should be able to handle it."

"That sounds fine to me," I said. "I know I'm going to be sore as hell, but I'd rather do it all at once myself."

I hung up the phone and suddenly had to sit down.

Oh, shit.

It was happening. Somewhere along the line, without my say-so, my life had taken a sudden and terrifying turn. I had navigated things as best as I could, and the attention I was getting from top specialists was inspiring and reassuring. But I was still terrified. It wasn't theoretical anymore; the appointments had been made, and I would be going under the knife—twice—in less than a week.

• • •

On Wednesday, I called Paul Pospisil, an old friend from my reporter days in Illinois. I hoped that Paul, a PhD chemist, former biotech executive, and current search firm partner, might be able to provide some insight on a question I'd been picking at since receiving my diagnosis: whether a positive outlook in the face of a terminal illness could measurably improve outcomes.

What I wanted to believe, and what I ended up choosing to believe, was that a strong general fitness level and a so-called positive attitude did indeed count for something in the fight against cancer; that the thoughts and prayers sent my way through thoughtful cards, emails, and phone calls *did* have some sort of healing power.

I'd first met Pospisil at a bar in downtown Champaign called the Esquire, my favorite spot to spend Thursday nights after my shift at *The News-Gazette*. Back then, Pospisil was a chemistry PhD student at the University of Illinois, but he was far from your typical "lab nerd." He enjoyed getting out to listen to live music, visit art galleries, and hang out at places like the Esquire, which tended to attract a diverse mix of townies, grad students, office workers, blue-collar types, and professors, all drawn to the comfortable atmosphere, legendary burgers, and free peanuts.

Since earning his PhD, Pospisil had worked for a number of biotech companies and was well-versed on cancer research and treatments. On the topic of whether a positive mental attitude was likely to be helpful in my cancer fight, he was his typically analytical self.

"Being positive matters to the extent that you have to pay attention and stay engaged in your own battle for survival to be successful," he said over the phone. "Those who have those good thoughts being channeled their way can at least fight their cancer knowing that they have that support. And I don't think you have to be religious to tap into this resource."

It turned out that Pospisil had a close friend who, like me, was fighting advanced cancer. "She talks to what she calls her higher self," he said, "asking herself questions about her situation and then working through the answers. She's learned not to let the medical process make her discouraged or lose heart."

"Makes sense to me," I said. "Whatever anyone says about the odds, I plan to work on not being dragged into negativity. And I know that's going to take a lot of work."

"That's the right call," Pospisil said. "You don't want to lose heart. And if you do lose heart, just let me know. I'll talk some sense into you."

• • •

Whether from the trauma or from the opiates, I can't remember large chunks of my hospital stay.

That's probably for the best; I think humans are wired through evolution to suppress traumatic events, and my hospital stay certainly was that. I *do* remember being terrified about undergoing a major shoulder surgery (with little to look forward to other than a kidney removal), but my fear was also the fear of the unknown that awaited me, which I knew would definitely include pain and suffering and which could very well include death.

I was wheeled to the operating room soon after my arrival. I don't even remember seeing Dr. Ferrone, though when I came to later in my bed and the anesthesia wore off, Katharina told me she had seen him just after the operation.

"He was sweating, but he said everything went fine," she said with a smile. "He looked like he had been working hard."

And in truth, according to the operation report I read later, my surgery proceeded smoothly with no complications. I was positioned in what the report called a "beach chair position" to provide access to my left shoulder and arm for Dr. Ferrone and the rest of the operating team.

The operation involved cutting into my upper arm along the humerus bone, then splitting my shoulder's deltoid muscles so a guidewire could be driven through the bone's center with an awl. This was followed by a humeral nail that was about thirty centimeters long. A locking cap was put on the top of the nail, and two bolts locked the nail in place at the elbow. My wounds from the surgery were then "copiously irrigated" (rinsed, in other words), my incisions were glued and stapled shut, and I was wheeled back to my hospital bed, where Katharina waited with Jakob and his girlfriend Ann.

The next day, Friday, was marked as a day of rest before my kidney removal on Saturday. At least, that was the plan; but it turned out to be a day of illness.

The first clue that something was amiss was my temperature, which kept creeping up. Lab tests followed, and after it was determined that I had caught a case of pneumonia, I was treated with Levofloxacin, a strong antibiotic. My temperature continued to climb, spiking at 101.7°F that evening. Suddenly, my surgery the next morning was in question.

"If your temperature keeps going up, we may have to cancel the surgery," Dr. Chang told me, when he checked in by phone to see how I was doing. "Hopefully the antibiotics will bring down the fever."

Thankfully, that's exactly what happened. By the next morning my temperature had eased down to 101.1°F, which Dr. Chang said was low enough to proceed with the nephrectomy.

"There's a slightly greater risk that you could get an infection," he cautioned, "but I'm pretty sure you'll be fine."

I had prepared myself for two surgeries in one hospital stay, and was worried about any deviation from that plan. "I don't feel that bad, actually," I said. "I mean, I'm sore and everything, but as far as I'm concerned, I'm halfway done. I just want to get it over with."

From what I recall of my second surgery, I met a doctor with a colorful surgical cap in the cavernous operating area. I was already sedated, still sore from my arm surgery and far from talkative. He asked me where I worked as he prepared my anesthesia, and when I answered Amherst College, he said, "No kidding! That's where I went to school."

Preparing to inject me, he asked, "How are you feeling? Are you ready for this?"

"I think so," I said. "You guys seem to know what you're doing."

"We like to think so," he said with a smile. A few minutes later, the radiologist reported that my pneumonia had begun clearing up, the colored-cap anesthesiologist gave the go-ahead, and that's the last thing I remember.

•   •   •

I woke up a few hours later and was wheeled to my hospital room. As my brain emerged from the fog of anesthesia, I realized that I couldn't move my right arm without feeling intense pain.

That can't be, I thought, still somewhat groggy. *My right hand is my lifeline. I need it.*

I was worried, but no one else seemed to be, including a resident surgeon making the post-surgical rounds. "Because of the way you were positioned on your left side during surgery, your right arm was lifted out of the way and past your head," he said. "It's possible that the long surgery time caused one of the nerves in your arm to stretch a bit."

The pace of my breathing quickened as panic flooded my brain. I pictured myself as a prisoner inside my own body, not being able to use either of my arms.

"That's my number one guess," the surgeon added. "The nerve being cut is unlikely; we didn't touch any area near there."

"How long will this last?" I asked. "I was counting on being able to use my right arm."

"Could be one day, could be ten days," the resident replied in a bored-sounding voice. "Hard to tell."

Great. Thanks for the sympathy.

He continued, filling me in on what I could expect over the next couple of days. It would take about twenty-four hours before I'd be able to take myself to the bathroom, but I could try walking the hallway of my floor the next day.

"You're going to be feeling some pain while you walk," he explained. "Your digestive system is kind of rebooting itself, and your incisions are still healing. It's important that you walk around, though. You need to be able to move around before we can send you home.

"Oh, and you look like someone who might overdo it. *Don't* overdo it. There's still a chance for internal bleeding."

Katharina, who was sitting in the chair next to me, raised her hand slightly to get the resident's attention. "I have a question," she said. "Peter has been working hard and now, all of a sudden, he's been diagnosed with Stage IV cancer. He's doing a good job trying to be patient, but he still gets really scared all of sudden." She was right about that; I'd definitely experienced a few anxiety attacks since everything began. "I've suggested that he call his doctor to see if he can get meds for anxiety," Katharina went on, "and he's been taking lorazepam as needed."

"Understandable, completely understandable," the resident said, nodding.

"But the nurses haven't been *giving* him the lorazepam," Katharina pointed out. "They're a little concerned about it mixing with his other meds."

"We will get him his lorazepam," the resident reassured her, and looked at me. "The main thing to remember is that the kidney removal was successful, the arm surgery was successful, you're looking good, you're sitting up, and you'll be walking soon enough. I'm as disappointed in the right arm as you are, but there's no reason to believe that it won't get better soon."

He nodded goodbye and left the room. I took a deep breath, thankful that Katharina had spoken up on my behalf. I *was* scared—scared about my diagnosis, my prognosis and the future. Lorazepam, also known as Ativan, had been helping dull the jagged edges of anxiety, especially as I lay awake at night trying to sleep.

That was the first time in my life that I had turned to anti-anxiety medication. More than four years later, I'm still an "as needed" user. Most days I don't need it at all, but when bad medical news arrives unexpectedly, or I have scans coming up and I can't shake my worry, I won't hesitate to reach for one of those round white pills. To me, the price I may be paying neurologically is worth it if I can avoid feeling some of the stress that research suggests can compromise immune responses.

● ● ●

I was discharged on a Tuesday, after a busy nurse gave Katharina a rushed lesson on wound dressing and dropped a large plastic bag containing assorted sterile gauzes, tapes, and medications on her lap. Katharina steered our car into the circular drive at the entrance of the hospital, and I walked slowly toward her, careful not to jostle my healing innards.

My right side and left shoulder felt like they absorbed every bump and sudden stop of the two-hour drive home. When we pulled into the driveway, our longtime friends Christina and Bob Furlone were waiting for us.

Bob gripped my right elbow and guided me up the back porch stairs, through the kitchen and living room, and helped me settle into the recliner that friends and family had chipped in to buy for us. Christina said it was this very model which had been such a lifesaver for her father after his major surgery, and in truth it greatly eased my recuperation.

The cinnamon-colored "Ultra Comfort" recliner was, to put it mildly, a motorized behemoth. It came with a remote that could raise, lower, and even lift me out of the chair, thus sparing my healing, sliced-through, and very grateful abdominal muscles the strain of getting up.

That first night I slept fitfully in the chair. Nearly every twist and turn hurt, so I stayed on my back and tried to relax. I can be a restless sort of sleeper, so it wasn't easy. My ultimate goal was to heal enough so I could climb the staircase that led to my bed, which I viewed as a significant marker in the return to normal activity.

I would also work to wean myself off the painkillers I was taking. In the hospital, I had pressed away without a care at the red button that delivered opiods intravenously via a Patient Controlled Analgesia (PCA) pump, frequently hitting the limits of my prescription. The operative motto was "Stay on Top of Your Pain," but now that I was home I wanted to spare my remaining kidney the extra work of filtering the pain relief meds, be it from ibuprofen or hydromorphone. I probably ended up enduring more pain than I needed to, but then again, I've avoided getting addicted to opioids—at least so far; I make no promises for the future.

Late the next morning, Jakob came to me bearing breakfast: a cup of coffee and a rice cake slathered with Nutella. I arched an eyebrow. He gave me an embarrassed grin, swallowed, and spilled the beans.

"It's actually not Nutella, dad," he explained. "Well...it *is* Nutella, but there's more to it than that. It's got weed in it, too."

Hmm, I thought. *I know he's just looking out for me. But on the other hand, weed's illegal. How's dad going to thread this needle?*

"Jakob, I appreciate you doing this and all, but you do know that marijuana is illegal, right?"

"Yeah, Dad, I know. But I really think it should be legal, especially for medical use."

I nodded. "Okay, I can see that. But how do you know it's going to work? How do you know you have the right dosage?"

"Relax dad, I did my research," he said. "There's all sorts of stuff online—recipes, videos, comments; everybody's got an opinion. I went for one that's pretty easy and that everyone seems to agree works. I melted some coconut butter, added the weed, and mixed it in with some Nutella."

He handed me the rice cake. "I really think you should try it," he added. "I think it will help you deal with pain, and it might even settle your mind, too."

I nodded slowly, acting as though I were carefully considering it. In truth I had decided to give it a try about halfway through Jakob's explanation, as my right side gave a painful throb. *Maybe the weed will give me some relief.* "Jakob, I appreciate you looking out for me," I said with only a hint of sarcasm. "I know I should say something disapproving about all of this, but I can't really get too worked up right now. In fact, I'm grateful. I really appreciate the trouble you went through to make this for me."

I paused. "I'm going to ask for a favor, though. Keep this quiet, okay? Your friends don't need to know that you're feeding me pot brownies. If you tell them, they'll tell their parents, and pretty soon it'll be all over town that the Rooney's are potheads. Keene's funny like that."

"Rice cakes, dad," he gently corrected me, "not brownies. And I'm not planning to tell anyone, even though I really don't care what people think."

I took the rice cake from his proffered hand and examined the brown mixture on it. "How much of this should I eat?" I asked.

"I'd start with a small dose," he said. "Maybe a quarter of the cake. It's hard to know what your tolerance is; everybody's different."

It was good advice. I should have followed it.

I did start with a quarter of a rice cake, using a kitchen knife to quarter the round slice into four wedges. I waited 15 minutes. Nothing. I ate another wedge. Fifteen minutes passed, and still nothing. I ate the third wedge. I waited 15 more minutes and nothing was happening. I eyed the last wedge.

"Jakob," I called. "I'm not feeling anything yet and it's been almost an hour. Should I eat the wedge?"

"I never said you should eat the other two," he reminded me.

It's true. He hadn't. But what did he know?

"I'm going to eat the last one," I said. "I'm thinking you didn't put enough weed in your mixture."

Fifteen minutes later, the first effects began to creep up on me, and pretty soon after that a stampede of sensations and feelings quickly unmoored and threatened to capsize my suddenly very wobbly consciousness. This intense trip was a far cry from the mellow buzz I thought I would be getting. Pure agitation swirled with high-octane paranoia to make me feel more trapped than I'd ever felt. I wanted to jump from the recliner and escape outside, but my surgically fragile body wouldn't allow it. I tried to remind myself that this would be over soon. I reached for reassuring thoughts: *Breathe deeply. Relax. This too shall pass.*

They helped a little, but not much. Closing my eyes was a mixed bag; at first the darkness would seem relaxing, but then my eyes would glimpse disturbing images, like wisps of creatures snarling and swiping at me. I blinked my eyes open and saw Jakob was already by my side, handing me a cup of water.

I sipped gratefully. I tried not to be mad at him for bringing me the weed.

You're the one who ate too much, I thought. *He's not the one who got impatient. He didn't eat the whole damn rice cake.*

●　●　●

Eventually, I fell into a feverish sleep and found myself in a strange dream, one in which I wasn't myself, but rather some sort of swashbuckling warrior. One hand brandishing a sword, I rushed down a fiery tunnel, stabbing at grotesque monsters that tried to wrap themselves around me. Surprisingly, this was no nightmare, and I wasn't scared. Instead, I felt strong and confident.

I sliced my sword through a monster's tentacles with satisfying squelches. I woke up just as I was prepared to finish off the monster with a mighty chop at its exposed, veiny green neck. I was breathing heavily.

My forehead was sweaty, but I didn't feel hot. Jakob was still on the sofa next to the recliner, calmly reading. I reached out and tousled his unruly hair. I felt more lucid and less high, but I was also calmer, more confident. *Maybe that warrior lives inside of me,* I tried to convince myself. *Maybe it can give me persistence, resilience, and courage when I most need it.*

I try to be sparing with the sorts of martial metaphors that are so often part of the cancer patient's perspective. Most of the time I don't really see myself as a "cancer warrior," but just another being in the infinite universe, living my life one day at a time. But the events of the dream *did* happen to me—they *did* feel real, even if it was fueled by eating too much Nutella-infused weed. I saw myself as a marauding cancer killer, successfully beating back the cancer beast.

I'm still able to summon that image of my life force in my mind's eye when I need it most. I've learned that cancer may never completely disappear. When and if it comes back, it feels good knowing that I've got a warrior inside of me that's going to fight hard to keep it at bay.

9 May You Be Mindful

The eight weeks I took off from work to heal served as a sort of temporal cocoon, one that protected me from the complicated world that crackled outside the confines of my home.

It was the first extended leave of my professional life. I had not taken any significant time off since I began work as a reporter on January 3, 1986. That was the day, just a few weeks before the birth of our first son, Max, that I drove forty-five miles from Champaign to Charleston to make it for the first day of my new job as a general assignment reporter at the *Times-Courier*.

Recuperation proceeded at its own pace, one sore step at a time. Katharina's sister, Gertrude, visited from Austria for two weeks. A former nurse, she and Katharina carefully changed my bandages, monitored the progress of my healing shoulder and right flank, and kept up my spirits.

Katharina was wonderful. She made sure to cook nutritious broths that were easily digested. We went on walks together, which started out embarrassingly short, maybe a hundred yards or so, gradually building up a little further each day. After a couple weeks, I added the occasional trot to test my right side, and my healing abdominal muscles were ready to withstand more strain.

Although the pain I'd felt during the first days back from the hospital was serious (probably a 6 on the 1–10 scale), after a week I had totally weaned myself off painkillers.

After two weeks, I was deemed sufficiently healed to begin radiation treatment. While the dosage had been determined by a radiology oncologist at Dana-Farber, the treatment itself was actually planned and carried out at Cooley Dickinson Hospital in Northampton, under the supervision of Dr. Jennifer Haider and her team. The radiation's purpose was to kill cancer cells—in the left arm and above the knee in my right femur where a bone scan had showed evidence of a small tumor, despite my feeling no pain or discomfort.

"The goal is to beat back the cancer in both areas," Dr. Haider said, "but we probably won't get rid of it for good without some other kind of treatment."

The radiation sessions lasted about thirty minutes total, and each left me a bit more tired. By the tenth and final session, I was seriously fatigued, even though I made it a point to walk for at least fifteen minutes each day.

• • •

I was thankful to have two more weeks following the radiation to recover before returning to work at Amherst, where much had changed during the eight weeks I had been gone. The snow had melted away, graduation was approaching that weekend, and the search for a new college president was well underway.

Our office staff was responsible for planning everything associated with commencement weekend, including writing, proofreading, and printing programs, escorting our honorary degree recipients around campus, and lining up sometimes hung-over seniors for the graduation procession.

Layered atop commencement weekend was a busy agenda for college trustees, who would be having their spring board meeting. I was expected to attend the meeting and offer input on issues as needed, but I expected most of my attention would be focused on making sure commencement weekend proceeded smoothly.

I climbed the worn marble stairs to my office in Converse Hall slowly, feeling a twinge in my right flank with each step. My left arm still felt more like a dangling appendage than a useful limb. As I went to open the office door, my mind was racing. I took a deep breath and settled down (a bit). I didn't *feel* very strong, but then I remembered that line from Woody Allen: "Eighty percent of success is showing up."

The first email I read that morning was from Susan. It was typically short: *Peter, welcome back. Kindly come to my office when you come in.* I walked down the marble stairs again and made my way to her office, knocked lightly, and entered when I heard her familiar call: "Come in!"

I settled into a chair across from her desk, careful to mask the discomfort I still felt. Susan's work load had only increased with my absence, and for that I felt somewhat guilty. At the same time, I wanted to demonstrate that I still could do the job, and take back some of those tasks. I wasn't ready to be put out to pasture quite yet.

During my absence, the search to replace outgoing President Tony Marx had hummed along, with interviews between finalists and members of the search committee taking place in discrete locations, such as airport lounges and hotel conference rooms. The process had yielded a finalist who had to clear one last hurdle: a meeting on campus with the trustees, basically a final job interview before a formal offer could be extended.

"We don't know when a formal announcement of her appointment will be made," Susan explained, "but I expect it will be soon after that meeting. We're looking for you to put a plan in place to announce her hiring."

How am I supposed to do that? I wondered. *I'm still sick from radiation and sore as hell.*

"No problem," I said, in as calm a voice as I could muster. "Who is she?"

"I'll tell you, but you can't let anyone else know," Susan said. "If word gets out about this before we're ready to announce, it's a fireable offense."

"Well, at some point others will have to know," I reasoned. "We'll want to interview her when she's here on campus. We'll want to interview members of the search committee and others who know her. We'll want to do all that in video, if possible. So I'm going to need help, which means I need to loop people in."

Susan nodded. "Her schedule is going to be very tight. Let me think about where we can do those interviews. There will be lots of students and parents wandering around campus for graduation."

"How about the president's office?" I suggested. "The backdrop is perfect, the location is good, and if we do it on Saturday there won't be many people in the building."

"That might work," she said. "Keep thinking about the details and the logistics. Get back to me with a plan by the end of the day.

"Here's what I can share on the candidate: her name is Biddy Martin, she's the chancellor at the University of Wisconsin in Madison. You can loop people in now if you think you need to, but I'd hold off until you get a plan together that I can share with the trustees."

In response, I asked, "She really goes by Biddy?"

Susan gave me a faint smile. "That's my understanding. Her real name is Carolyn, but all anyone ever calls her is Biddy. It's a nickname from her childhood. You'll need to double-check that, though."

"I'm on it," I said and slowly stood up.

Susan looked at me with some concern. "I know you've been through a lot. Are you sure you're up for it?"

"I think so," I said. "I'm going to find out, I guess. And I've got some good people to help me out."

"Well, make sure to take it easy, if you can." She said and gave me a sympathetic smile. "It's good to have you back."

●   ●   ●

The resumption of my professional life, along with my hour-long commute, gave me plenty of time to let my mind wander. Being newly diagnosed with advanced-stage cancer, it tended to wander toward places rife with agitation.

It was worse at night. As my mind raced, I thought of pain, suffering, and death. I worried about Katharina, Max, and Jakob, and how me dying of cancer would affect them. I also worried about myself. How would I handle this journey? Would I be dignified and courageous, or terrified and cowardly?

To cope, I first turned to my chill pills, the Ativan I had been prescribed shortly after my diagnosis to cope with anxiety. Benzodiazepines like Ativan work by slowing down communication between the nerve pathways in the brain, and a .5 milligram pill at night always settled me down enough to fall asleep. I didn't reach for a pill every night. It depended on how my day had been and how strong my underlying worries were that night. I wasn't proud of needing a pharmacological support, and I respected the addictive nature of this drug class. As a result, I tried to be sparing in my use of this drug.

During the day, exercise was my stress reliever. As the days since my surgery and radiation slipped by, my walks became punctuated by longer stretches of running, while the pain in my right flank continued to subside.

I tried to vary my exercise routine to maximize my recovery. If it was raining outside and the Amherst pool wasn't too crowded, I would take to the water, grabbing a flotation belt from the equipment shelf and "walking" vertically through the water, stroking my arms in various patterns to expand my range of motion. Progress was slow, but within a few weeks I was swimming again, first the breast stroke, then a few crawl strokes, and then a few back strokes.

•   •   •

Colleagues like Caroline Hanna, the media relations director; Katie Fretwell, the dean of admissions; Betsy Cannon-Smith, the alumni secretary; John Carter, the chief of campus police; and Marcus DeMaio, the college's videographer, helped keep me motivated and encouraged me with their unwavering support during this period of rehabilitation. I remain grateful to them.

At home, my illness had jolted both Katharina and Jakob, and they expressed it in different ways. For Katharina, the events of the last three months had been traumatic. It's hard to see the bright side of terminal cancer, and her mind often jumped to worst-case scenarios. Whenever it did, I tried to cheer up both of us with a mental game I called, "It Could Be Worse."

The way it worked was, each time her mind came up with a worst-case scenario, I would concoct a what-if that was far worse. "I could have had children later, meaning they would be toddlers now instead of young adults that I had been fortunate enough to raise for many years." "I could be without medical insurance." "My doctors could be clueless." "My cancer could be even more aggressive than it seemed to be."

Yet no matter how often I thought of my blessings, there were still times that I felt overwhelmed by stress and anxiety.

Jakob, feeling the stress as well, had decided to quit the varsity volleyball team midway through its spring season. He was also having difficulty waking up in time for school. I suspected my diagnosis and treatment had unsettled his world, though he didn't talk about it with me directly.

Instead, he dealt with the anxiety he was feeling by turning to mindfulness meditation, attending meditation sessions at a center in downtown Keene. He didn't tell me he was doing this until a few weeks after he began. We were hanging out and watching TV when he brought up the authentic peace he found sitting on the floor with other adults, concentrating on breathing and clearing his mind.

"I think it's helping me," he said. "I've been getting worried about a lot of things, and this kind of helps me deal with that."

Jakob didn't open up very much or very often to me, so I was elated that he had chosen to do so. I proceeded cautiously, not wanting to ruin the moment." I'm really glad that meditation is helping you deal with things, Jakob," I said. "I know it hasn't been easy for you."

"Maybe it would work for you, too," he suggested.

I couldn't really see myself sitting cross-legged on the floor with my eyes closed, surrounded by strangers. I didn't have anything *against* the notion; I just couldn't imagine having the patience for it.

All the same, I was intrigued. I'd met a couple of professors at Amherst who were deeply involved with mindfulness, and had incorporated contemplative practices in their own courses. I was willing to give it a try.

"I'm always looking for ways to deal with stress," I admitted. "As you can imagine, I worry about how things will turn out for me and for all of you guys. Any suggestions?"

"Well…" Jakob began. He glanced at me quickly then looked away before continuing. "Basically, if you focus on your breathing and nothing else, you can deal with stress better. We spend a lot of time doing that—just sitting around and breathing. Also, there's this guy at U-Mass named Jon Kabat-Zinn. He wrote a book about dealing with stress called *Full Catastrophe Living*." He gave me sheepish smile. "Umm…if you want to listen to his book, I have it downloaded. He's also recorded some meditations. I can get some of those for you if you want."

Thus began my introduction to mindfulness, courtesy of the soothing voice of Jon Kabat-Zinn reading from his best-selling book, *Full Catastrophe Living: Using the Wisdom of Your Body and Mind to Face Stress, Pain, and Illness*. In the book, Kabat-Zinn provides the underpinnings for the eight-week long Mindfulness-Based Stress Reduction course that he pioneered at the University of Massachusetts Medical School.

Kabat-Zinn has been a leading figure in the mindfulness movement, which continues to find adherents by offering a way to dial back the stress of our busy lives by helping to develop the capacity to pay attention to moments that would normally avoid conscious notice. Meditation offers a way to bounce along on the waves of life with equanimity, and maybe even help calm the waters. It sounds simple, but it is not easy, Kabat-Zinn cautions. It takes serious commitment combined with a spirit of non-striving, a difficult trick to pull off.

It all starts with cultivating mindfulness. The beginning premise, Kabat-Zinn explains, is that no matter what is wrong with you, as long as you are breathing there is more right with you than wrong. Though stress is an unavoidable part of the normal human condition, and facing our problems is the only way to get past them, there is an art to facing those problems, one which involves embracing the change that we have no control over while realizing that it is *not* a disaster to be alive, even if we might be facing adversity. Just because we are feeling pain and suffering doesn't mean we shouldn't also open our minds to the possibility of joy.

The phrase "full catastrophe" in the title refers to the protagonist in the novel *Zorba the Greek* (later played by Anthony Quinn in the movie) who, when asked by the narrator whether he has ever been married, answers loudly, proudly, and with great gusto, "Have I ever been married? Of course! I have a wife, kids, the full catastrophe!"

Zorba's reply is not meant as a lament, as Kabat-Zinn is quick to point out, nor does it mean that having wife and kids is a catastrophe. Instead, Zorba is expressing appreciation for the richness of life and the inevitability of all its dilemmas, tragedies, ironies, and sorrows. So-called 'full catastrophe living,' as Kabat-Zinn sees it, is a call "to laugh in the gale of catastrophe and to never be weighed down by the sorrow of defeat for long."

Both the book and Kabat-Zinn's voice on my iPod were reassuring tonics for my soul at a very vulnerable and difficult time. Kabat-Zinn offered a simple definition for the practice of meditation: he referred to it as "paying attention, on purpose, to the present moment." Unlike prayer (or my conception of prayer, at least), meditation doesn't involve asking for anything. It's all about acceptance and non-striving, bringing your mind away from thinking about the past or the future.

Among the lessons that I absorbed from Kabat-Zinn's writings was the notion of letting things unfold at their own pace, without trying to rush things. To illustrate this point, Kabat-Zinn describes a child trying to speed up the metamorphosis of a caterpillar to a butterfly by opening up a cocoon, killing the insect in the process. Striving is discouraged and acceptance is encouraged.

For me that often seemed incongruous—why wouldn't I want to strive to cure my cancer? Why would I want to accept my diagnosis and fate? Upon reflection I realized Kabat-Zinn had a point, though it is important not to confuse acceptance with resignation, or even worse, surrender. Instead, non-striving and acceptance were ways to avoid the mental anguish of obsessing over what might have been or what should be instead of focusing on what is.

Kabat-Zinn's lessons on breathing were also extremely helpful. As he explained, a foundation of being mindful is the ability to concentrate on one's breathing, to be aware of it without thinking about it. This can help us cope with stress, agitation and restlessness.

The basic gist of mindful breathing is this: we are diaphragmatic breathers when we emerge from our mothers' womb; our bellies expand as we inhale and contract as we exhale. Somewhere along the way, this natural rhythm gets lost. If we learn to focus on breathing this way again, even for a minute or two at a time, we can make great strides in relaxing ourselves and addressing stress. Breathing in this way—gently exhaling and inhaling through the stomach, slowly yet deliberately--provides a way to counter the surface agitation of one's thoughts. It let me dive into my mind's deeper recesses, where things were calmer and not nearly as unsettled.

On those nights when sleep was hard to come by, whether due to an upcoming medical appointment or a pain in my chest, listening to Kabat-Zinn would settle me down.

My mind would still wander, of course, and I'd still find myself asking whether I would ever find the courage to accept my situation if it should deteriorate, or be able to treasure the remaining moments I would be given. But eventually my mind would settle, my breathing would relax, and I'd drift off to sleep as Kabat-Zinn's meditations resonated through my earbuds and the moments slipped away until tomorrow became today.

10 Can the Mind Heal the Body?

Jakob, with his quiet, contemplative manner, had led me to meditation and mindfulness and its potential to mitigate stress. It was his older brother Max who reminded me that relentless focus and a positive attitude were also effective ways to deal with life's most challenging moments.

Max had found the perfect outlet for his outgoing, gregarious personality. Since his junior year at the University of Vermont, he had been working for Northwestern Mutual, a financial services company based in Milwaukee. In the two short years since he had graduated, Max had emerged as one Northwestern's top representatives--in part because of the long hours he was willing to put in, but also because of a personality that genuinely enjoyed the company of others and the challenge of persuading prospective clients from all walks of life that it was good for them to set aside money for retirement, life insurance, and other financial products.

The job had its challenges, the biggest one being that it was purely commission based, and Max frequently felt insecure in his ability to continue producing at the level his bosses expected him to.

"There are some days that I just don't feel like calling anyone to set up meetings," he once said during one of his frequent calls to me. "And if I do set up a meeting, half the time they blow me off. It's frustrating."

"You know what I do when I don't feel like dealing with people?" I said. "I do something else that needs doing—there's always something. For me, that might be writing a story for the college website or editing someone else's work; for you, it might be paperwork that you've been putting off. Even extroverts like you need a break from people."

I'd had my own experience with sales in college. In my case, it was selling advertisements for the yellow pages of university phone directories—way back in the days before Google, when every student, faculty, and staff member would be issued a campus phone book. The job took me all over, calling on pizza parlors, tanning salons, book stores, ice cream shops, and any other businesses that targeted students.

To my surprise, I was good at it. I still remember my biggest sale to the manager of printing and copying services at Northwestern University. He'd been evading me for most of the summer and finally agreed to see me toward the Friday before my last week in town. The meeting went quickly. I showed him what he'd ordered the year before, threw a few ideas at him, and he'd re-upped and then some inside of ten minutes. It was quite a way to end the week for a college student. I still remember coming back to the Holiday Inn where we staying, ordering a drink, and heading to the pool for Friday Happy Hour, laughing and enjoying the summer afternoon with colleagues and newfound friends.

In Max's first year as a financial advisor, while he was still in college and working as an intern, Katharina and I agreed to be among his first customers. It took my son, during one of his first sales presentations, to remind me that there was something to be said for life insurance, even if, like most people, I was skeptical of its value and resentful of the bite it took from my take-home pay.

Years earlier, long before Max had become a Northwestern Mutual representative, I had been pinned down by a persistent Northwestern agent who had persuaded both Katharina and me to buy whole life insurance and disability insurance. At the time I couldn't really imagine needing either product, but once again an agent's patient salesmanship had carried the day.

While I decided to cancel the whole life policy a few years later and convert it to a cheaper term policy once I began paying Max's college tuition bills, I kept the disability policy. Amherst

College also offered long term disability for all of its employees, a benefit amounting to 60 percent of annual pay. I also knew from my research online that Stage IV kidney cancer was a special category which qualified for fast track approval with Social Security. In the meantime, Max assured me that Northwestern would more than likely approve my claim. So if my cancer grew or the side effects of the treatment became intolerable, it looked like we would be able to get by. Chances were pretty good that I wouldn't have to go gangster, "break bad," and resort to cooking meth in the backwoods of New Hampshire to pay for my cancer treatment and make sure my family was provided for if I ended up dying.

Of course, Max scoffed at the notion that I'd ever even need to file a disability claim. "Don't be talking about disability, Dad," he said, during one of our frequent phone calls." You're going to be working for a while because you're going to kick cancer's ass."

"Well, we'll see what happens," I said. "I know I'd be very lucky if that were to happen."

"It will happen, Dad. You just have to believe it hard enough and it will happen."

This was more than just wishful thinking on Max's part. At the time, Max's life philosophy was one which appreciated the value of focused, positive thought.

This mindset was conveyed to me in a heartfelt email he sent to me late one evening:

> *Dad,*
>
> *When I talked to you tonight, you made a comment that made it sound like you would be "lucky" to totally recover or beat the cancer. I can certainly appreciate that it may feel this way, hopefully only for a fleeting moment or two, but I don't ever want you (or any of us) to ever believe that or get in the habit of thinking that way. I don't care what the odds or statistics say. The power of believing transcends that. If I let my mind or natural human tendency get the best of me on a regular basis, I would have failed out of my business years ago; as all of the odds and statistics are against me by about a 95% chance of failure. I know that your*

odds are much better than that, especially if you believe. Look at what you have done so far: having an awesome marriage, family, career, etc., all starting at such a young age. What are the odds of that? Everything that you have done in your life up to this point makes beating cancer look like a piece of cake. I need you to be strong. I will be strong, too. We all will be strong.

Max had singled out something—namely, dogged persistence—that was working for him, and which had certainly worked for me in the past. It was a trait I had always valued, but one which seemed to be in conflict with the non-striving nature of meditation.

• • •

Yet persistence is part of my nature, just as it is part of Max's. Maybe that's why I began incorporating guided visualization exercises into my wellness routine, and the soothing voice of Jon Kabat-Zinn began to compete with the folksy, rumbling Texas twanged baritone of Gerald White for airtime on my iPod.

I'd first come across White on ACOR, the Association of Online Cancer Resources, which is a platform for patients and caregivers to ask and answer questions about all aspects of this frightening disease. Every type of cancer had its own listserv, or online discussion group, and the kidney cancer group is especially active. (ACOR has since become SmartPatients, an online community where cancer patients and caregivers learn from each other about treatments, clinical trials, the latest science, and how it all fits into the context of their experience. I highly recommend it.)

When the topic of guided imagery first appeared on the ACOR discussion thread, I was skeptical. But after seeing some rational voices weigh in with support and testimonials, I decided I had little to lose beyond the forty-five dollars that White, a long-term survivor of Stage IV kidney cancer, was charging for his book and CD. *Three Months to Life* is White's account of his victory over cancer through relaxation and guided imagery, and the CD it comes with visualization exercises White developed and which he credited for putting his cancer into long-term remission.

I certainly won't claim that guided imagery has healed me; I know that the likelihood of a long-time remission, to say nothing of a cure, is a day-by-by proposition. Yet, looking back, there have definitely been times when listening to White's gravelly voice describing white blood cells in battle with cancer cells was just what I needed.

"There's never been a type of cancer or cancer cell that a healthy immune system could not kill in open combat," he says on the CD, the haunting tones of Navajo flute music echoing lightly in the background. Quoting the physician and philosopher Albert Schweitzer's remark that "there's a doctor inside of every patient ready to be called upon to help with healing," White notes that every cancer cell has on its surface an antigen (short for antibody generator) that the body's different types of white blood cells can identify and kill.

"I rarely ever meet a patient who's ever even heard of a neutrophil, a macrophage, an NK cell, or even a T cell," White's sonorous voice would intone through my earbuds as I listened to him night after night, waiting for sleep to come. "Yet these are all friendly-yet-deadly fighters, present in the human immune system and ready to go to war with cancer cells."

The goal of his guided imagery exercises was to train the subconscious right side of the brain, which controls the body's involuntary responses, such as getting the lungs to breathe, the heart to beat, or the immune system to fight disease, to respond to suggestions coming from the brain's left side.

These exercises in visualization, in which I imagine my various white blood cell types taking on and conquering my cancer cells, may have played a role in whatever healing has happened. More importantly, these exercises have helped me relax when sleep is hard to come by. They've provided me with at least the illusion of having some control over my body's immune system and its ability to conquer cancer, perhaps not forever, but long enough to keep it at bay for a few years.

To enlist the power of the immune system, White claims that patients should first better understand—so they can then better visualize and then enhance—the crucial role that the various white blood cells play in keeping them healthy. "There's even a scientific name for this: pyscho-neuro-immunology."

If stress and fear are the accelerators on the road to death, White asks, then what are the brakes? "The answer to this question is relaxation, pure and simple," he says, encouraging listeners to take deep breaths, slowly and deliberately." Letting the breath out through slightly pursed lips, one can then go a step further by thinking of words 'breathe in hope, breathe out fear,'" he adds.

White's discussion of visualization also deals with positive mindsets to promote hopeful outlooks: "Our first objective will be to rip out the old wiring of despair and replace it with new wiring of information-based hope."

Before that can happen, however, it's important for cancer patients not to get hung up on the question of "why." As in, "If our immune systems are so good at fighting cancer, then how did the cancer get into my body and spread in the first place?"

"This is a question that leaves many patients unable to proceed, but I think it has an answer that is so simple, that it seems to have gone unnoticed," White says. "The answer is that it didn't get in, as from an external source like a germ does. No, it was born there as a mutation of good cells, and dwelt unrecognized among the friendly cells.

"It is unreasonable for even the best guard dog to recognize treason in the mind of a family member until it exposes itself," White continues. "In the case of cancer in the human body it is not unreasonable to assume there is a threshold of recognition based on the health of the immune system, below which cancer cells can sneak in under the radar screen. In far too many cases, far too much collateral damage has occurred before the antigen recognition occurs, if it occurs at all, and thus death becomes the outcome."

White also suggests that cancer patients listening to his CD set themselves visual goals, such as witnessing a child's wedding or graduation, or some other significant event. Doing so, he says, will enlist the subconscious mind which "must be continually reminded that its objective is to deliver you alive and well to that remembered event, when its place arrives in the chronology of real time."

Thanks to White, I allowed myself to be optimistic again, visualizing my body's white blood cells killing cancer cells like Pac–Man munching on power pellets. For many days, as I listened to his voice night after night, I found that I was able to shed some of my anxiety and find a place in my mind where hope could triumph and where I could visualize a path for stability and remission.

11 A Cancer Warrior Fights Another Battle

Years later, shortly after my initial meeting with Gordon Freeman, I had the opportunity to speak with Gerald White by phone. He'd agreed to discuss his guided imagery work, while I intended to thank him for his contribution to my healing and well-being. I wasn't prepared for the latest dramatic twist his life had taken—at the age of eighty-three, twenty-two years after his initial diagnosis, White was coping with a cancer recurrence in the form of a golf ball–sized tumor in his right lung, discovered while being treated for a sepsis infection.

Gerald White was fatigued but polite and gracious, patiently answering questions that he surely found to be tiresome, having been asked them so many times before.

I, like many others, wanted to hear his thoughts on what is essentially an unanswerable question: is there any proof that visualization works?

White's deep voice spoke a tad more slowly than on his guided imagery CD. He seemed philosophical and thankful for the lengthy respite cancer had given him.

"There's something I should tell you about this recurrence of mine," he said. "I say this with no pride at all, but after all those years of enjoying a free life, I finally cut off the imagery. There were about five years there where I didn't keep to it. And I'm the guy who wrote the book, right? Then we, quite by accident, found this resurgence, so I blame myself for a lot of this. I just relaxed. I thought the battle was over, and it wasn't."

Now, White said, he not only listened to his own CD, he and his wife also offered a prayer for healing each time he took one of his "cancer pills." He also listened to a CD with prayers spoken by his grandsons years ago, during his first fight with cancer.

Back then, he had his left kidney removed, along with the massive tumor inside it. The cancer recurred in the renal bed and subsequently spread to his lung. He then underwent an early form of immune therapy that involved injecting himself with Interleukin-2, a type of antibody meant to stimulate the immune system. He was on the treatment for about eight months, and remembered with revulsion being sick for most of that time.

"It was like the worst flu I ever had in my life, and I had steady tumor growth the whole eight months," he recalled. "I finally just said, 'The hell with this; this isn't living. I'm going to solve this problem on my own.' I just walked away from it."

White spent the next few months researching the notion of whether meditation, prayer, and guided imagery could stimulate the immune system.

"If you go back in time to 1993, there just wasn't anything for kidney cancer," White explained. "Now, people are trying targeted therapy drugs and God knows what. I just knew I had to come up with something else, because they weren't going to do it. I told my doctor if medical science can't solve this problem, then engineering science will, because I'm not going to die from it. I made good on that. I completely cut off the IL-2 treatment."

Spending hours in local libraries and consulting the works of noted experts like Herbert Benson, Frank Lawlis and Carl Simonton, White said he developed his own guided imagery exercises and soon became cancer-free.

"Three months later, I went to the same oncologist," White recalled. "He put the films up and said, 'Well I'll be a son of gun,' except he used a word other than gun. He said, 'I don't know where your tumors went, but they ain't there no more.'"

After his cancer went into remission, White became an outspoken advocate for kidney cancer patients, serving a three-year term on the Kidney Cancer Association Board before developing a patient mentoring program for the University of Chicago, which he then directed for about two years.

As White told me his story, my rational side reminded me that as powerful as his story was, there was also the possibility that he had experienced a delayed reaction from the immune therapy treatment he had been receiving just a few months before his cancer retreated. I asked him for his thoughts on this observation.

"'Delayed reaction' is the comfortable answer," he retorted. "That makes everyone comfortable. That means 'Let's discount it completely.'"

"I'm not saying discount it completely," I quickly answered. "I'm saying that maybe you can't single out one particular thing. It could be a combination."

With irritation in his voice, White answered, "Maybe I can explain it this way and you can understand it: I didn't feel my mission was to peel back the foreskin of science. I just wanted to get well."

We both agreed that seeking out the best possible medical care is a must for anyone fighting cancer. So is being willing to go outside medicine and within the depths of our own subconscious mind to fully engage in the battle.

"We call this complementary medicine," he said. "It's meant to augment the best technology and medicine you can find."

White said he's never understood why medical researchers aren't more interested in studying long-term survivors like him, to perhaps unlock a path to healing that would work for more patients. "They use terms like anecdotal, which is a name they give to something they can't explain," he said. "Medicine has the luxury of doing that. Engineering doesn't. We can't dismiss something as being anecdotal. If a wall comes down and kills someone and we say it's anecdotal, that doesn't help us a lot. I had a doctor tell me that my survival was anecdotal. And I said, 'Well, I'd rather be a live anecdote than a dead statistic.'"

White estimated that about 2,000 people have tried his CDs, and that about 300 have achieved some sort of remission while doing so.

"There are very few that didn't at least get something out of it—partial remission, or extension of life; if nothing else, at least a good night's sleep," he said. "I've had a lot of people come up to me and say, 'You're the first person that was able to help me put away the fear enough so that I could sleep.'"

There's no way to specifically credit the program in a way that would hold up to the rigorous protocols that medical research demands, and that, White said, is one weakness of medical research today—an unwillingness to harness or even study the power of the mind to heal.

"The whole basis for many clinical trials is to minimize the placebo effect," he said, referring to the documented phenomenon of having a fake treatment (usually an inactive substance like a sugar pill or a saline solution) improve a patient's condition because he or she has the expectation that it will be helpful. "When I was on the Kidney Cancer Association Board, I stood up at many a meeting and said, 'I don't understand—one of us is using faulty mathematics here. You're saying if you see a response of forty percent, you want to make sure it's the effect of your drug and not the placebo effect. I'm saying, 'Why not take whatever we can get from the placebo effect and add it to what we can get from the drug and come up with a bigger number? Why not kick a nineteen percent response rate up to almost forty if you can get that much from the placebo effect?'"

White says physicians would counter with the basic sentiment that he wasn't being scientific. "I would say, 'I'm probably the only person here who has practiced the scientific method, which can be expressed by two words,'" he said, and there was a pause on the other end of the phone. "Do you know what they are?"

I muttered something along the lines of forming a theory and then setting out to try to prove it.

"Observing and inferring," he said. "The great scientists are those who can make numerous observations and infer why that may be. It never was very complicated. I saw what happened in my own case, and from that, I inferred that this damn stuff can be beat."

White stressed that he was not bitter, but deeply appreciative of the extended survival he had enjoyed. As we finished our conversation, he left me with one thought: "You know what's going to happen? I'm going to die one of these days. It's been a great run, and if you think I'm complaining, then you've got the wrong impression."

Gerald White passed away in August 2016 at the age of eighty-five. He did indeed have a great run. He devoted decades of his life to help others cope with cancer and to find hope and courage within themselves.

That might not be enough, in and of itself, to cure cancer. But getting a decent night's sleep, along with a respite from anxiety and worry, isn't a bad consolation prize, either.

PART II
Finding the Path

12 When the News Isn't Good

On the drive into Boston, I could tell that Katharina was as nervous as I was. It was just a year after my initial diagnosis, and a break in the usual routine had us both on edge. For the first time since all this began, there'd been no news from my most recent CT session. And no one in my situation put much stock in the adage "No news is good news."

I'd had bone scans and CT scans twice in the past year. It had become something of a routine: driving to Dana-Farber, parking the car, and heading to the original Dana-Farber building's basement, where most of the imaging took place. On our way there, we'd walk past the pediatric cancer wing and catch glimpses of children surrounded by family members with love and worry evident in their eyes. Empathy would flood my brain whenever I saw them as my focus switched from myself to others. I would realize all over again how cancer ravages indiscriminately.

The radiology waiting room only reinforced that sense of randomness. Patients looked like card players in some cosmic casino, playing hands that varied greatly. Plenty of people looked perfectly healthy, but there were always a few in rough shape, gray faces sucking oxygen through tubes, careworn eyes looking at the floor.

Everyone was waiting for some sort of imaging, be it CT, PET, MRI, bone, or x-ray. All the tests were scheduled, conducted, and evaluated here by a talented team that had their craft down cold.

Each time I showed up for a scan, I made sure to inform the staff members that I was missing a kidney and nursing a sore shoulder with a titanium rod hammered through my humerus. That way they knew to check my creatinine levels and adjust their contrast dye dosage accordingly. Contrast dye is known to be hard on the kidneys, but without it, the tumors would not pop out to the radiologists viewing the images.

The radiation these tests exposed me to was also a concern; I've had CT scans every three months for the last five years, and the cumulative effect of so much radiation carries its own health risks. But when you have Stage IV cancer, you learn that there are a lot of these types of trade-offs, where the side effects of treatment can be so bad that it would be perfectly reasonable to forego them altogether, in favor of a higher quality of life. (I'm not judgmental about people's treatment decisions, and I hope they respect my treatment decisions, as well. We're all in this together, after all, and no one gets out of here alive anyway.)

In terms of risks vs. benefits, CT scans can catch tumors when they're still small, at the point where treatment can be most effective. But despite their excellent imaging detail, a chest CT scan also delivers about seventy times more radiation than one chest x-ray, according to the American College of Radiology. There's even research suggesting that figure may be *under-estimated*; that CT scans might deliver *hundreds* of times the radiation of x-rays, possibly increasing the risk of cancer from CT scans alone.

Yet most oncologists treating Stage IV kidney cancer patients recommend quarterly scans, scaling back the frequency only if the patient has had no recurrence for two years or more. So I and the other patients in the imaging waiting room shared the unsavory duty of swilling down our two plastic bottles of a barium-sulfate solution (now available in banana or berry!) which helps to generate better CT images.

Speaking again on the topic of benefits vs. risks, drinking this chalky liquid would usually result in a case of the runs, which kicked in shortly after my scans. I'd head straight for the luxurious bathroom on the first floor of Dana-Farber's new Yawkey Cancer Care Center, and after a digestive system purge, I'd pop a tab of Imodium in the hopes of stopping things up.

After that, Katharina and I would drive back home, overshadowed by a sense of dread that would last until I heard the results. If I wasn't careful, I'd visualize the wrong thing—images of cancer cells darkly expanding, munching on and poisoning healthy tissue.

Luckily, cancer caregivers know about this anxiety, and the considerate ones will share scan results by phone or email, especially if the news is good. Dr. Choueiri was that type. No more than two days after my first scans were taken (about four months after my surgeries), I was nervously awaiting the results when my cell phone rang. I had only to see the 617 area code of Boston to know it was a medical call.

"Mr. Rooney, it's Dr. Choueiri," his melodic voice said. "I have some very good news."

"That's great to hear," I said. "What news is that?"

"Well, things are much better than we expected. I'm looking at the pictures now and I see no evidence of disease."

Relief and a deep sense of happiness washed over me. I savored the feeling, breathing deeply, but it wasn't long until I felt the first twinge of concern. I can't help it; I'm a worrier. "And has the radiologist written a report?"

"Not yet, at least not that I've seen. But I would be surprised if his conclusion is different. I think you should be happy. Call your wife, enjoy the news together."

I could hear the hum of a workplace in the background, and knowing that Dr. Choueiri juggled clinical work with a busy research schedule, decided not to keep him busy answering a hundred questions. I thanked him for taking the time to call me and, after confirming that I should still come in for my Thursday appointment that week, said goodbye. After I hung up, I reminded myself to savor the feeling of elation that had accompanied the good news and not immediately look to the future with worry.

As my mind wandered inevitably from the present, I slowly allowed myself to feel more optimism about my future. Maybe I *was* actually making headway against this disease, not through any treatment, but through my own determination and a grab bag of approaches that seemed to be working for me, including meditation, visualization, cancer-fighting supplements such as curcumin, and regular exercise. My path forward seemed clear: aim to kick-start my immune system, quit worrying about the future, and just try to live in the moment.

Three months later, another positive scan report followed the first one. Once again, I allowed myself to think about the future a little more optimistically. As green grass bristled up through melting snow, I was tempted to proceed with the plan we'd discarded with news of my diagnosis, that of moving down to Amherst to buy a house in the small yet vibrant college town, with its mix of rowdy college students and opinionated townies and easy access to nearby Northhampton and the other interesting communities that comprised the Pioneer Valley of western Massachusetts. While homes there were definitely more pricey than in Keene, avoiding the psychic toll of my daily hour-long commute would make that price difference worth every dollar.

Following my latest scans, though, there had been no phone call from Dr. Choueiri. No friendly voice informing me that the scans are terrific—amazing, really, showing no evidence of further disease.

I tried to rationalize it optimistically. *He's a busy man. I can't expect him to call me with scan results every time. The fact that he did so at all was a huge favor. He certainly doesn't have to. But…*

I wonder if it means something.

●　●　●

I was getting used to making it through the gauntlet of traffic that surrounds Dana-Farber and the dense cluster of real estate that encompasses Boston's Mission Hill neighborhood and the Longwood Medical Area. Just down Brookline Avenue from Fenway Park, the Longwood area employs thousands, from brain surgeons to custodians.

The neighborhood includes institutions such as Simmons and Emmanuel colleges, Northeastern University and Harvard Medical School, several hospitals like Boston Children's, Brigham & Women's, and Beth Israel Deaconess Medical Center, research institutes like Dana-Farber and the Joslin Diabetes Center, and biotechnology and pharmaceutical company offices such as Merck Research Laboratories.

All of which made me realize, as I turned left on Jimmy Fund Drive to head into the comforting underground cocoon that is the Dana-Farber parking lot, how lucky I was to live within a two-hour drive of this epicenter of medical care and commerce.

After we parked, an elevator brought us up from the depths to the tenth floor, where huge windows offered commanding views of the busy city to patients waiting for their appointments in cushioned chairs. Small refrigerators and cabinets were loaded with snacks and beverages, and there were even iPads available to borrow.

After my name was called, I followed a nurse's assistant to a small booth, where she took my blood pressure, weighed me, and sent me back to the waiting area. After a few more uncomfortable moments in the waiting area's comfortable seats, my name was called again, and the nurse's assistant led Katharina and me down a hallway to an examining room that still looked new.

As we were entering, I heard sounds from a nearby room and glanced down the hall. A doctor was leaving an adjacent examining room, followed by a man and a woman who looked to be in their fifties. Their pace was slow, and they wore stunned expressions, as though they were still absorbing bad news. They walked slowly past us while the doctor disappeared down the hall, his white lab coat receding along with the brisk tap-tap sound of his shoes.

We sat in our room for a few moments, nervously eyeing our sparsely appointed surroundings, which included little more than an examining table, a desktop computer, and cabinets. Then there was a quick rap, the door opened, and Dr. Choueiri entered. He closed the door behind him and consulted his notes.

"Well the labs are good, and we'll talk about that," he said after a brief greeting. "But the scan *did* show some growth this time. Not in the bones, the bones still look good, but in the lungs. There are lung nodules that had been stable and now are growing."

I was stunned. *Lung nodules? What happened to "no evidence of disease?"*

"They're extremely, *extremely* small," Dr. Choueiri emphasized. "But these aren't really a candidate for surgery, because there are a number of them. There are some that have increased from four millimeters to six millimeters, and from five to seven millimeters."

Katharina and I didn't say anything. Dr. Choueiri seemed to be leading toward something, likely the answer to the question which remained unsaid: *What now?*

"There's also one around the spleen, too small to be noticed two scans ago, though in retrospect you can see it there," he continued. "It's still extremely, extremely small, but it's there. About half an inch."

"On the spleen?" Katharina asked.

"Near the spleen," he corrected. "I'm not worried about that one, not at all. These aren't major changes. That said, it *is* more than the last two scans. So the question is, what to do now?" He looked at us with his dark brown eyes before answering his own question. "As I see it, there are three options," he said. "One is to redo the scans in three months, see how these are growing. They're very small, and there's a chance they won't get much bigger. Option Two says we go on to some form of treatment--for example, Sutent or Votrient."

We'd discussed Sutent and Votrient before, and I'd spent some time researching them and reading about their effects online. These so-called "targeted therapies" worked by blocking chemical messengers from sending growth signals to cells, thereby stopping cancer cells from growing and dividing. They essentially cut off the blood supply to cancer cells, but the side effects in doing so could be quite severe, including elevated blood pressure, extreme fatigue, and something called hand-foot syndrome, a sort of itchiness and sensitivity that made walking and other tasks painful.

Needless to say, I had what could be called an irrational anxiety about these drugs, probably because of the side effects. The way I saw it, and there were plenty of patients who'd had a great run on both meds who disagreed with me, these drugs only bought you time—perhaps a few months, a few years if you were lucky—until the cancer cells devised a workaround and began spreading again. I was also convinced that exercise was helping my immune system keep my cancer at bay without any treatment, and these drugs were known to make exercising difficult.

All this meant that I was reluctant to consider this treatment as anything other than a last resort. So, naturally, I was quite interested to hear about option three.

"Option Three will be to try what we call High Dose Interleukin 2," Dr. Choueiri said. "This is a treatment we do very rarely, and only at Beth Israel.

"The issue is that only a very small number of patients actually benefit from HDIL-2. But you are the type of patient who might— no heart disease, excellent kidney function, minimal disease anywhere else. Patients like you can at least have a discussion on whether or not to do this."

I already knew a bit about HDIL-2 from the online support group. The treatment had been approved by the FDA in 1992, and was offered primarily to kidney cancer and melanoma patients due to the fact that those cancers don't respond well to chemotherapy. From 1992 until 2005, when Sutent and then other targeted therapies first gained FDA approval, HDIL-2 was the only mainstream treatment option for treating Stage IV kidney cancer.

I also knew how rough the treatment could be for the patient. HDIL-2 requires an extended hospital stay, during which lab-manufactured antibodies are pumped into the patient, kick-starting the immune system so that it can hopefully identify and kill cancer cells. It doesn't work for most people.

But it cured a few.

Dr. Choueiri looked at me, then at Katharina. "Those are the options. We could try removing them with surgery, which might work for a time, but they will grow back. This isn't one lesion."

Even as he said it, I couldn't help but picture the small tumors in my lungs, growing slowly but surely to consume everything they touched.

"I can email one of my colleagues at Beth Israel and tell them that you are an optimal candidate," Dr. Choueiri offered. He was trying to make me feel special, though I certainly didn't feel like it. There's not much to like about earning first prize in the cancer contest.

"What do *you* think?" I asked. *He's the expert, after all.*

"I think you should go and at least hear about the HDIL-2. That is the only potentially curable option that we have right now," he said, pulling out his smartphone. "I can email Dr. McDermott right now. What do you think?"

"I've read that HDIL-2 has an eight percent response rate," I replied.

"That's for everyone," Dr. Choueiri pointed out. "That statistic includes patients that have heart disease, or who have disease growing everywhere. If you select only those candidates who have the best chances, the odds are much better. One study reported a twenty-two percent response rate. I think you should hear about it and the side effects."

I asked a few more questions—how much work would I miss? How many lung nodules do I have? How long after treatment do you know if it's working? And even as I asked for specifics, I thought about the question I *really* wanted answered. *What do I have to lose? If it can cure me, it's worth a try, even if the odds are low and the side effects are bad.*

While Dr. Choueiri typed out an email to his colleague at Beth Israel, Katharina looked at me and said, "Better the lungs than the brain."

"Absolutely," Dr. Choueiri agreed from his computer.

"You really don't check the brain, do you?" I asked.

"We really don't," he replied. "Not unless the patient shows symptoms. We do one baseline, which we did a year ago, but we really don't check again. Though," he added, "you'll probably need another brain MRI before starting HDIL-2."

He finished, pressed send, and looked at me.

"We're going to beat this. You have to believe that. So hang in there and be positive."

With that, he left the examining room. Katharina and I looked at each other and followed him out the door, each lost in our own thoughts, trying our best to follow the doctor's advice as we made our way down to the parking garage.

As we did, I couldn't help wondering how we looked to anyone passing by. Did we look like that other couple, faces frozen in shock, trying to come to grips with the turn their life has taken?

HDIL-2: The Original Immuno- therapy

One thing I keep reminding myself about cancer is that it's a numbers game.

Twenty-two percent doesn't seem like a very encouraging number. Just think: if someone told you there was a 22 percent chance of rain, would you carry an umbrella or wear a raincoat before heading outside?

Odds are, probably not. But cancer patients like myself often need to turn relatively low odds around in their heads, seeking a way to justify rolling the dice anyway. It kind of comes down to options and what makes sense given your own unique situation. In my case, I was looking for some HDIL-2 patients who might have come through hell and ended up on the other side.

It didn't take long to find them. At that time, before ACOR updated its platform and rebranded itself as SmartPatients, the kidney cancer listserv was a no-frills, searchable online message board. It was then, and remains to this day, full of valuable information. The board is moderated by Robin Martinez, a widow of a kidney cancer patient who has made it her life's mission to preside over a welcoming, informative, and quackery-free zone of support and comfort to cancer patients and their caregivers.

As long as dialogue is respectful, no topic is off limits. Posters can seek advice about treatment, health insurance, and end-of-life decisions, while others can write about the 'scanxiety' they feel, or else describe another cruel visit from the Beast, what many of us called cancer.

The next morning, I sent out a query with the following subject line on ACOR:

"Should I Try HDIL-2?"

I had nine responses to my question within a few hours. All of them advised me to take a chance on HDIL-2, despite its tough reputation, because it offered a chance for long-term remission or even a cure. One user, Randy, wrote that he'd received three rounds of HDIL-2 over seven months more than two years ago, and his status was NED—No Evidence of Disease.

"The treatment is tough, but if you can get it, it can work," he wrote. "I'd be happy to share my experience, and my wife can share the experience of the caregiver—a different and critically important role—if you'd like. We wish you the best and send prayers. Fight Hard!"

Oliver wrote from the perspective of a partial responder. He had been stable for more than five years before his mets began growing again.

"The Votrient is holding the mets stable and it has been for over two years," he wrote. "I am seventy-two years of age and looking forward to many years of continuing health and activity."

Calling herself an "eight-year NED responder, thanks to HDIL-2," Peggy offered an enthusiastic endorsement for the treatment. She described her situation when diagnosed: a large tumor in one kidney and tiny mets, too numerous to count, all over her lungs.

"After failing a clinical trial and before becoming symptomatic, I started the HDIL-2 program in UCLA," she wrote. "My response after the first two week-long sessions, and a short rest period, was 'significant shrinkage' to the largest of my mets, and within four months, all were gone.

"I was fifty-five at the time, had been anemic due to the cancer for over a year, a few months out of surgery, and NOT athletic. Now I am healthy, active, walk over two miles three to five days a week, travel, and hope that patients get all the information about all the options, including HDIL-2, early in the treatment process."

Caroline, another complete responder, wrote, "IL-2 is tough on both the patient and your family. However, we all knew that going in. Probably the most important thing you can do beforehand is talk to other people who have experienced it and encourage your family to talk to other caregivers, too.

"Looking back, I think the most important thing is to have the support of your family," she concluded. "Also, please allow yourself to recover fully before rushing back to employment."

Then there was Vicki, who wrote the following simple response from her iPhone: "YES!!!!!!"

These were the types of responses I was looking for to help my inner optimist fend off my inner pessimist. At various time during the previous year, that optimist had successfully urged me to feed off of the positive energy of friends, family, colleagues, and fellow cancer patients. Heeding its voice, I had often prayed, not to God but to the cosmic force of the universe and its potential power, to hear and respond to calls for healing. I reminded myself that I wasn't a statistic; why shouldn't I be one of the lucky few who respond?

My inner pessimist weighed in: *You were screwed by the odds already. Only 3 in 10,000 get kidney cancer, so what makes you think you can beat the survival odds? Just deal with it—you're probably going to croak in a few years.*

It was a continuous struggle to find an authentic attitude of hope without too much worry that would allow me live in the present and get my mind in the right place.

And where was that place?

For me, it was a mental state of acceptance without anger, and a spirit of determination, not passivity, in waging this campaign against cancer. It was a quest to be brave in the face of adversity, to keep in mind the words on the Tibetan prayer flag that hung on the porch at the home of our friends Christina and Bob Furlone. It read:

Courage
    Not the absence of fear or despair
    But the strength to conquer them.

14 In Good Hands

When the time came for Katharina and I to head out for my first appointment at Beth Israel Deaconess Medical Center more than a month later, I had decided to go forward with the HDIL-2 treatment…provided I passed medical muster.

Katharina supported my decision, even though it would mean a lot of sacrifice on her part. After all, if she even wanted to visit me during my hospitalization, she'd be stuck finding a place to stay in a city where a good deal on a hotel room still meant $250 a night.

Beth Israel is located on Brookline Avenue, just a block south of the Dana-Farber buildings. After I checked in and filled out the various forms required of new patients, a nurse guided us to the examining room. On the way, she informed us that we would be meeting with Dr. James Mier, who was part of the team that administered HDIL-2 and who had been doing it since he first started conducting clinical trials on it in the late 1980s.

A few minutes later, there was a soft knock on the door and a young woman entered, also wearing the requisite white lab coat. She introduced herself as Alexandra Bailey, an oncology resident who was part of the HDIL-2 team.

Dr. Bailey sat down and began asking me questions about my medical history, but it didn't take long before I was the one asking questions. The first one to tackle was about the tumor that had developed near my spleen.

"Doesn't the spleen produce white blood cells?" I asked. "It seems kind of ironic to have a tumor develop right next door to the cells that are supposed to be killing cancer cells."

Dr. Bailey quickly corrected me. "Actually, it's the bone marrow that produces the white blood cells. But you're right; the spleen *is* an immune system organ. It functions to filter the blood and help with infection response. That said, I don't think there's any kind of significance to having cancer near or even on the spleen."

After asking me for a bit more information about my symptoms and whether I felt they impacted my daily life, she launched into an explanation of the HDIL–2 treatment timetable.

"Week one, you're being treated," she said. "Week two, you're off. Week three, you're being treated. Four weeks from then, weeks seven and eleven, is when you'll get scans. We scan twice because the body's response to this treatment is often delayed.

"The second round of this treatment would be scheduled after you came in to see us at week twelve, which is three months after you started. Then, if there is benefit observed on *those* scans, we talk about doing the whole thing again."

"What's the percentage of people who re-scan?" I asked.

"In general, IL–2 has a low percentage of people with a substantial response to treatment," she admitted. "If you add up the number of people who have a complete response, meaning the cancer goes away, or partial response, meaning it shrinks by thirty to forty percent, those numbers are generally in the twenty-five to thirty percent range.

"What we've tried to do here," she said, "is screen for those people who are most likely to have a better outcome. Younger people, people with clear cell carcinoma, which you have, people who do not have any brain involvement, people who are overall more fit and healthy. People with lung involvement also tend to do better. As a result, our response rates here are higher than the national average, which is about ten percent."

All of this sounded encouraging to me, but as Katharina was quick to remind me, I wasn't selected for treatment just yet.

My next question was one I had been asking most of my doctors since my journey began: did Dr. Bailey (and by extension, her team) think there was any evidence to suggest that factors like having a positive attitude, meditating, or practicing visualization improved the odds of beating cancer?

"My opinion is that it does help, though randomized clinical trials can never be done to ascertain the extent of the benefit," she said. "Still, it's my belief that your attitude does make your body better able to tolerate treatments and better able to get treatments that are going to kill your cancer."

"To be honest, I never really got sick until I was diagnosed with cancer. So I feel like I *do* have a fairly strong immune system; it just needs to be told where these cancer cells are."

Dr. Bailey nodded." On the other hand," she said, "if you don't respond to HDIL-2, I wouldn't say it's because of your attitude or the particulars of your immune system. I can't even say what it is about one person's cancer that makes them respond or not."

"You'd have a higher response rate than twenty-five percent if you could," I said.

"Much higher," she agreed.

•   •   •

Dr. Mier came in a short time later. I stood up to greet him, looking into the eyes of the man who was largely responsible for developing and fine-tuning the treatment that I now hoped I would soon be undergoing.

Dr. Mier wore a white lab coat over a shirt and tie. His hair was graying, and his eyes were slate-colored and tinged with blue. He shook my hand, then Katharina's, and sat down.

"So, I understand that you and Dr. McDermott have been doing this treatment for quite a while," I said, starting us off.

"I was doing it when Dr. McDermott was in high school," he said with a laugh. "This is my project. We have probably treated a thousand patients since we started doing it back in '86."

"So, if you were in my shoes, would you do it?" I asked.

"Yes, of course," he said. "I wouldn't even hesitate."

"Even though there still a lot of mystery as to who will respond and who won't?"

"It's still a complete mystery," he agreed. "There is no predictable biomarker for the benefit. There are some features that help us predict good or bad outcomes; we are very fond of lung metastases, for example."

Dr. Mier explained that the human body's immune system varies considerably from location to location. "There's a whole system that protects the gastrointestinal tract, for example, completely different from the system that protects the lungs. There are cells that will only hone in on one particular area of your body to eradicate an infection, clear a virus or, as in this case, clear out cancer."

According to Dr. Mier, the exact mechanism by which HDIL-2 fights tumors remains unknown. Thankfully, physicians now know to administer antibiotics during the treatment to counter the possibility of developing a staph bacterial infection (usually from the insertion into a vein of the line that delivers the treatment to the body.)

"Even though HDIL-2 therapy is an immune stimulant, it actually interferes with the part of the immune system that deals with bacterial infections," Dr. Mier admitted. "If you read early papers on HDIL-2, there was a four percent mortality rate on the treatment; you had a 1 in 25 chance of dying."

Obviously horrified by such a high mortality rate, Dr. Mier and the other clinical researchers sought to zero on its cause. They found that the infection rate was far higher than in similar procedures, such as inserting stents or pacemakers. This led them to wonder whether the treatment was hindering one part of the body's immune system while stimulating another.

"We found that the neutrophils, which are the white blood cells that deal with bacteria, become completely functionless during HDIL-2 therapy," he said. "A lot of the fever and chills that looked so much like infection was, in fact, infection. Untreated, it probably contributed to the death of those patients on the early years. That simple decision to put everyone on antibiotics eliminated that problem altogether. As a result, we've almost completely eliminated the mortality associated with that."

Another major modification to the treatment involved keeping patients in the hospital for an extra day after the last dose had been administered and testing their blood to check for a rheumatic, fever-like illness which causes inflammation of the heart.

"What happened—again, this is twenty-plus years ago—is we'd send someone home and he'd die of a heart rhythm problem. Patients who developed this problem had no chest pain, no presenting symptoms. But now, if we find they have this abnormality, they're put in cardiac care for a little longer, and we keep everybody an extra day. That eliminated that problem."

The final major development, Dr. Mier said, was the realization that it took a team of dedicated nurses carefully monitoring patients during the entire process to stay on top of the side effects, such as fevers, chills, shaking, nausea and diarrhea, that still occurred.

"That accumulated experience is very important for the nurses who actually deal with the patients on a day-to-day basis," he explained. "We doctors are kind of the least important part of the equation."

With that, Dr. Mier began describing the treatment I would hopefully be receiving.

"You'll be getting an infusion of an antibody called Proleukin[3]," he said, "which is a man-made protein that performs the same action as native human interleukin-2. Interleukins, by the by, are the messengers by which white blood cells communicate with each other to coordinate inflammation and immunity. Among its actions, IL-2 increases the number and activity of certain types of white blood cells—namely T-lymphocytes, or T cells. In fact, before IL-2 got its interleukin designation, it was originally titled 'T cell growth factor.' It has the ability to sustain the growth of T cells once they're primed with a foreign protein, what we call an antigen. The T cells become responsive to HDIL-2 and actually expand in numbers."

Basically, the body produces interleukin naturally when faced with a bacterial infection. HDIL-2 floods the body with laboratory-made interleukin to stimulate the growth of T cells, in hopes that the T cells will recognize and kill the cancer cells.

"Your body is receiving a genetically engineered version of interleukin in amounts that you would never make on your own,"

---

3 Proleukin is made by a company called Prometheus, which became a part of Nestlé *Health Science* in 2011.

Dr. Mier said. "That way, we can hyper-stimulate the immune system to do things that it was never really designed to do."

"So why doesn't the treatment always work?" I asked.

"Because there's no guarantee that a tumor has anything that even remotely interests the immune system," he said. "There's nothing foreign about them for the immune system to pick up on."

"And there's no other treatment at this point that is as promising or has as much potential?"

"Not without being needlessly hard on your system," he replied. "There *are* some newer immune therapies being investigated that are looking rather promising, but here we have the advantage of decade-long observation periods, where positive initial responses are shown to be permanent."

The other challenge with the newer immune therapy clinical trials, as Dr. Mier explained it, was the extremely limited amount of space available to patients. "Depending on how promising the drug is, those slots could be gone the day they're announced," he said. "It's like a rock concert that everyone wants tickets for; they can come and go in no time at all. Plus, until something is FDA approved, you have no control over it."

"Does this treatment shut any doors for me, in terms of clinical trials down the road?"

"Virtually none," he said. "It's one of the only treatments where that's the case. If you were to go on just about anything else, all sorts of doors slam shut. IL-2's about the only thing you can give to someone and then come back with the investigatory agent later on, including some of the other immune-based therapies."

I made sure to ask him about the side effects of HDIL-2, and how debilitating he expected them to be.

Dr. Mier's answer was reassuring." The body makes IL-2 on its own, after all; it's a natural product," he said. "You're just getting a genetically engineered version of what you make every time you have the flu. It's no more of a drug than insulin is. You're just getting it in more abundant amounts than what you can make on your own. When you're ill with the side effects of HDIL-2, all sorts of things can go awry. But it's all reversible."

In fact, Dr. Mier said, while most of his patients chose to rest during the week-long break between their treatments, some of them chose to go back to work. "Now, those are the outliers, and in all honesty I don't recommend that," he added. "But you get over the different side effects fairly quickly. The fatigue lasts a while, as does the dry skin, but your appetite generally comes back even before your start your second week. Some people will experience diarrhea during the first week, but often just the gap between the final dose and your discharge time is enough for that to resolve."

"Thanks so much for your patience in explaining this to me," I said. "Is it safe to say that, for someone with my prognosis, things aren't as dire as they were five years ago?"

"Not as dire, no," he agreed. "If you read the old literature, the majority of people died within a year of their diagnosis. But that hasn't been true for years. I think it's reasonable to shoot for a complete response out of this so you can live normally."

And with that, he had persuaded me.

"Well, I'm willing to give it a try, I guess," I said. *Besides,* I thought, *it's not like I'm full of other options.*

•   •   •

We said our goodbyes, and a short time later the nurse who'd escorted us returned. She introduced herself as Nancy Weinstein and told me she'd be taking care of scheduling my preliminary appointments.

Before I could begin treatment, I would need to have an MRI of my head, a CT scan of my torso, an exercise stress test that tested pulmonary function, and an EKG to ensure that my heart was up for the treatment. She then she gave me an overview of what I could expect from a typical week of treatment:

"When you arrive on Monday, you'll meet with a nurse practitioner who's going to oversee most of your care that week. Her name is Virginia Seery. You'll then meet Dr. McDermott, who's the attending physician that week, as well as the surgeon who will put your central line in. That's done hopefully by mid-day, and the line goes in at the bedside.

"Then you'll get an x-ray to check the placement of the line. Once that's all set, the orders and lab work is drawn, and the order goes down to pharmacy for the drug to be made. The first dose is given at 4:00 pm, after which it's given every eight hours, assuming that all things are good to go.

"It only takes fifteen minutes for the drug to go in. Once the drug starts going, you'll then need to have a continuous infusion of IV fluids. You won't have to worry about eating, but you're welcome to eat if you want to. That said, you shouldn't worry if you don't have any appetite; your appetite will likely decrease as the week goes along. If you have any comfort foods you'd like to bring in, you're welcome to do so."

"Does that include comfort beer?" I asked.

"Comfort beer, no," she said, giving me a smile.

She then went over the side effects:

"Oftentimes, the first side effect is shaking and the chills, what we call rigors. Your job as a patient is to tell nursing when you're beginning to feel a side effect, whether or not you're beginning to get a little shaky, or a little nauseous, or whether or not you have a sore. None of this stuff will go away without a drug.

"In other words, we can't help you unless you tell us," she noted. "This isn't the time or place to suck it up and grin and bear it. It does *not* happen that way. The nurses all know you're not just whining, so don't worry.

"As the week goes on, you'll be getting more and more fatigued. Odds are you'll start thinking about how much you just want it to be over and done with. We want that for you, too, but we also want to get those doses into you. Communication is a two-way street. If you've been having a rough time and not sleeping, then you can negotiate and say, 'You know what, I need to skip the midnight dose so that I can make sure to get two doses the next day.' That happens. So you have to talk."

Another unpleasant side effect was that I was going to become bloated with water weight from the IV fluids I'd be receiving. The extra water would disappear within a few days of going home, she said, but while I was at the hospital I would probably gain fifteen to twenty pounds.

"The HDIL-2 tends to put these micro-holes in your capillaries, which means water from your blood is leaking out," Weinstein explained. "When the blood volume decreases, that means your blood pressure decreases. In order to get your blood pressure back up, we give you more fluids. We're kind of chasing our tails, but while that's going on we may be giving you boluses of 250–500 ccs of fluid."

Finally, she mentioned that during the second week of treatment, my bed would be alarmed, meaning I couldn't leave it without help from one of the nursing staff. The reason for this was apparently due to my becoming more unsteady as the treatment wore on.

"So, what do you think?" Weinstein asked, as she concluded her overview.

"I think I'm up for it," I said. "It sounds pretty grueling, but if it works, it's worth it."

"It *is* grueling, but we've been doing this for a while. If I don't see you before your treatment, good luck."

With that, she left the room. Katharina and I followed her soon afterwards, each of us lost in our own thoughts. Mine were still a bit garbled, trying to process everything I'd been told, trying to visualize a positive path through the treatment, hoping that I'd be part of minority who responded well to treatment.

• • •

A couple of weeks later, after completing all of the tests that Weinstein had described, I was sitting in my office at Converse Hall when my cell phone vibrated. I saw the 617 area code and picked up.

It was Dr. Mier.

"Peter, I'm just calling you to let you know that we've hit a little roadblock," he said.

"Oh…really?" I said, trying to keep the sudden dread out of my voice. "What is it?"

"I'm looking at the report of your brain MRI, and there's a very small lesion; tiny, really. I think we can clear it up quite nicely, but it does mean that your HDIL-2 treatment will have to be delayed until we take care of this."

15 Brainiac

When I heard the words 'tumor' and 'brain' in the same sentence, my stomach tried to twist itself in half. I stood up, more than a little unsteady, and closed my office door.

"I'm sorry, Dr. Mier," I said. "Can you repeat that?"

"I'm calling to let you know that you won't be coming in on Monday for treatment after all; you'll need to get this brain lesion treated first. But it's a tight little tumor; one treatment should take care of it."

"Does this mean I can't get HDIL-2?" I asked.

"This is a delay, Peter, nothing more," he said in a soft voice that I tried hard to find reassuring. "It won't change our plans. Sure, it used to be that if you had brain metastases, then you couldn't get HDIL-2 at all. Now we just zap them, make sure they're gone, and get you started on the treatment."

Dr. Mier explained that about ten percent of advanced kidney cancer patients develop brain tumors. In many cases, the lesions are isolated occurrences, treated while they are still small, and don't spread rapidly, but some of them do spread. In my research, I came across a poignant blog post titled *The Enemy Returns* and written by a history instructor from New Hampshire who had also undergone HDIL-2 treatment.

His pre-screening had also revealed a brain tumor, and he developed even more brain tumors after his treatment. His blog ended abruptly, but I was able to determine that he had passed away at the age of forty-one, leaving a wife and three young children behind. Another vibrant life force, ravaged by cancer's brutality.

"Okay," I said. "So what happens next?"

The next step, as he explained, was to meet with the neural operations team to schedule a procedure using a tool called a Cyberknife. Despite the name, it's actually a dose of highly focused radiation aimed straight at the tumor that kills the cancer cells without damaging the surrounding tissue. Three to four weeks after that, I'd get an MRI. If everything looked good, we'd be back on track. I'd go in and start my treatment as if nothing ever happened.

And for once, things played out according to plan. A couple of weeks later, I found myself lying on a cold long table in the basement of Beth Israel Deaconess Medical Center, my head inside a form-fitting mesh mask that was bolted to the table.

I wasn't quite feeling comfortably numb, but I was fairly relaxed thanks to a half-pill of lorazepam and focused breathing exercises. I'm not extremely claustrophobic, but a procedure like this one has the potential to make anyone feel a bit constrained. I listened to "Dark Side of the Moon" through earbuds connected to my iPhone and just tried to stay calm.

Meanwhile, a team of radiation therapists manipulated a whirring robotic arm from a nearby control room that delivered a high-powered beam of radiation to a five millimeter by four millimeter tumor on the left side of my cerebellum, a procedure which took about forty-five minutes.

Though my situation was sobering, I told myself that it could always be worse. I had been fortunate that the HDIL-2 screening had revealed the small lesion, located in the part of my brain that controls coordination, thinking, and personality, before it had grown bigger. The typical protocol, I recalled Dr. Choueiri telling me, was to scan the brain once after a Stage IV cancer diagnosis, and not again unless one becomes symptomatic through headaches, blackouts, or other neurological disorders.

I experienced no side effects from the Cyberknife treatment itself, other than a mild headache that I occasionally felt toward the back of my head, especially at the end of a long workday.

Still, I worried about my kidney cancer crossing the blood-brain barrier, and whether the HDIL-2 treatment would be able to do the same. Dr. Mier reassured me that the HDIL-2 still had the potential to be effective. He pointed out that my disease was stable elsewhere and that if my body *did* respond to HDIL-2, it would prevent future metastases from migrating to the brain.

• • •

As soon as my brain MRI was finished, it was officially the weekend for the Rooney's. Katharina, Jakob, and I left the hospital and headed north out of Boston to meet with my older sister Kati and her husband Jim, who had flown in from Chicago. We then all made our way to a rustic Maine cabin belonging to Christina and Bob Furlone. They were the ones who had arranged for the purchase of the "zero gravity" recliner which had allowed me to recuperate from my dual surgeries the previous year, and it was at their suggestion that we headed up to visit them at their property on the shores of Lake Aziscohos in the hilly woodlands of western Maine.

It was the perfect respite from the uncertain and daunting medical experience that I faced. Instead of hospital beds, there was a wooden dock where we could lay out at night to watch countless stars and the occasional comet shimmer brightly against a pitch-black sky, far from any man-made light sources. During the day, we explored the shores of the lake, picking up driftwood and swimming in the cool freshwater.

Suggesting a late afternoon cruise, Bob steered his boat along the lake before anchoring it in a cove where massive boulders jutted out of the inky water like the breaching backs of massive grey dinosaurs. As I dove off one of the boulders and plunged into the water, I pictured my body's cancer cells sloughing off of me as I swam underwater, holding my breath as long as I was able.

After two days at the camp, we said our goodbyes to the Furlones and drove the scenic roads of Maine, northern New Hampshire, and Vermont before eventually arriving in Burlington to visit Max. His job as a financial advisor at Northwestern Mutual had him working most evenings and weekends, but he still took the time to hang out with us.

It was a beautiful summer day as we headed to the park along Lake Champlain. I took along a Frisbee for a session of catch with

Katharina, Max, and Jakob, savoring the feeling of being together with my family.

In the afternoon, as the boys lounged on the grass beneath the shade of a maple tree, I slipped away to call Boston.

My goal was to get out of keeping my appointment in Boston the next morning, where I'd be informed about the results of my brain MRI. The appointment would mean several hours on the road to get information that could easily be conveyed by phone or email. Eventually, I was put through to Dr. Erik Uhlmann, a neurologist who kindly agreed to share my results.

"The MRI shows slight scarring that is consistent with the procedure you had last month," he said. "I think that you will be fine to proceed with your HDIL-2 treatment."

And so my long weekend was safe. Medical matters could be put on hold for a few days as Jakob, Max, Katharina, and I enjoyed each other's company and did our best to avoid any talk about doctors, cancer, and my upcoming treatment.

16 Toxic Treatment

I thought I was well-prepared for my first day of HDIL-2. Dr. Mier and Nancy Weinstein had both thoroughly explained the whole treatment process, and the hospital had sent an information packet to ensure that I was fully aware everything.

Even more helpful were the members of the online kidney cancer support group who had written about their treatment experiences. One line from those posts distilled the essence of what was soon to come: "It's like the worst flu you've ever had, times ten."

My room on the eleventh floor of Beth Israel's Reisman wing overlooked Brookline Avenue. If I looked out my window to the right, I could just see Fenway Park. Katharina and I had arrived at about 10 am, and we had more than enough time to get settled in. I had brought along some photos, which I taped to the wall in front of my hospital bed. One showed me approaching the finish line of triathlon I had entered two years earlier; another depicted Jakob playing trombone in his middle school band; another showed Max on his graduation day at the University of Vermont, flanked by me and Katharina.

These images were my reminders of why I was undergoing this ordeal: so that I could rid my body of this cancer and enjoy a longer life with my wonderful family.

Or at least make it until Jakob's graduation from college. Which means four years living with Stage IV cancer.

It seemed like a lot to ask for, but on the other hand, if one is to hope, why not hope big? I remembered a poem by Emily Dickinson, one which had been painted on a walkway mural at Brigham and Women's Hospital, along with depictions of birds of various types. I had passed it several times the year before on my way to appointments with Dr. Steven Chang, the urologist who had removed my right kidney.

Hope is the Thing with Feathers

"Hope" is the thing with feathers –
That perches in the soul –
And sings the tune without the words –
And never stops—at all –
And sweetest—in the Gale—is heard –
And sore must be the storm –
That could abash the little Bird
That kept so many warm –
I've heard it in the chillest land –
And on the strangest Sea –
Yet—never—in Extremity,
It asked a crumb—of me.

Emily Dickinson had been born in Amherst and wrote many of her poems in the bedroom of her house not far from Amherst College, where her father had been treasurer. It wasn't until after her death that her poems became widely known, her reputation blossomed, and her fiercely original reflections on human existence and nature were disseminated.

Compared to her, my own thoughts about my life were much more pedestrian, and touched more upon the chaos in all things, from my health to the weather. I looked out the window of my hospital bed and noticed a summer rain shower was quickly darkening the roads and sidewalks below, turning an overcast day into a slick and glistening slice of urban life, full of puddles, slashes of rain, and people huddled beneath umbrellas, swiftly walking toward their destinations.

The forecast for that morning had called for a "slight chance" of rain, about ten percent. Roughly the same odds as a positive, complete response from the HDIL-2 I was about to subject myself to. As I watched the scene below, it occurred to me, not for the first time, that what I was hoping for from HDIL-2 was a rare downpour of unanticipated rain.

During the early afternoon, I met with Virginia Seery, the nurse practitioner who supervised the nursing team on the HDIL-2 unit. Thin, blonde, friendly, and compassionate, she introduced herself with a smile. She had brought along a consent form for me to sign that succinctly listed, for the umpteenth time, the likely, possible, and rare side effects associated with the treatment—fever, chills, fatigue, rash, nausea, diarrhea, abnormal liver and kidney function, low blood pressure, heart muscle damage, inflammation, abnormal heart rhythm, fluid in lungs, infection, confusion, death.

I signed it all away, as Seery explained that I'd receive my first dose of interleukin in the late afternoon or early evening, after a brief surgery to place the line that would deliver it to my body. That happened about an hour later, when Dr. Nicholas Tawa entered my room carrying an assortment of surgical tools wrapped in plastic and gauze.

"So what I'm here to do," he said, after ripping open the packages he needed, "is to run a PIC line to your heart. It shouldn't take very long."

I watched him warily as he slid latex gloves over hairy hands and approached me. He eyed me from above his surgical mask. "What do you do for work?" he asked, and pushed a button on the bed's control panel to recline me below horizontal, to the point where I felt I was about to slip backward.

"I work at Amherst College," I said, now staring at the ceiling.

"No kidding," he said. "My son looked at Amherst. He ended up going to Tufts, though. Plays for the football team," he added proudly. "Keep very still," he added before applying a local anesthetic to my left chest. He waited a moment and then inserted a needle there, pushing my chest as he searched for the vein that would lead to my heart. On his third and final try—"If this doesn't work, we'll have to take you downstairs," he told me—he found the vein he had been seeking.

Blissfully, the poking stopped.

"Well, it looks like we've got it, but it'll take an x-ray to make sure," Dr. Tawa said as he took his leave. "It was nice to meet you."

Two hours later, an x-ray taken at my bedside confirmed that I was ready for my first dose. The bolus arrived, looking just like any saline drip bag. The only difference was this one cost $12,421.98. (I discovered this weeks later, after perusing the itemized bill for my 6-day stay. It amounted to a grand total of $133,941.06. Of that, I was responsible for paying $250, thanks to my health insurance plan through Amherst.)

I didn't feel any side effects from this first dose, or the one that followed. It wasn't until dose three the next morning that they began to kick in; fairly gently at first, with chills. I called for the nurse, who came in and covered me with two warmed blankets. When my face started to itch, Katharina applied some lotion to it.

My symptoms looked normal to Dr. David McDermott, who stopped by that afternoon. I had read about Dr. McDermott online. He was a prolific researcher, and patients spoke highly of him. If Dr. Mier was optimistic and sunny by nature, the dark-haired doctor seemed very serious. But, as Katharina noted later, "Cancer is very serious."

Dr. McDermott assured me that my side effects were well within the normal range. In fact, he informed me that I was a dull patient after checking my chart.

"Dull is good," he reassured me. "We like dull."

By my fifth dose, administered at midnight, the chills had evolved to rigors, and my whole body began to shake uncontrollably. The warm blankets were supplemented with a 50cc injection of Demerol into my IV line. The relief it brought was instant and welcome—an immediate cessation of the shaking and a leaden slumber that lasted for a few hours.

By Friday, I had absorbed eleven doses. Not as many as I would have liked, but as many as Dr. McDermott felt was safe. As had been predicted, my heart rate had accelerated to twice its normal rate while my blood pressure had dropped dramatically. I had experienced some vomiting and diarrhea, but no mental confusion.

I was determined to get up and move, so twice a day I put on a robe and, pushing along my IV pole, would shuffle around the eleventh floor. I would usually stop by a lounge at the end of the hall, where patients undergoing treatment or their visitors could rest in recliners that overlooked the city.

During my week off from treatment, I rested both at home and at Spofford Lake, where Katharina and I belonged to a sailing club. It was there that we pursued our recently acquired hobby of racing Sunfish boats. But there would be no sailing for me this week. Instead, covered in blankets despite the warm weather, I reclined in the shade and watched the sailboats tack back and forth, seeking the swirling breezes that agitated the surface of the lake.

•   •   •

By the end of my week of rest, I was feeling much better. I still wasn't looking forward to my second week in the hospital, and I was especially dreading the insertion of the central venous catheter. It was nothing personal, but I hoped Dr. Tawa wouldn't be doing the procedure again.

My hopes were quickly dashed. His hairy hands rooted around inside my chest once again, though this time he found the vein more quickly. Katharina held my left hand during the procedure, and that calmed me down.

"What a way to spend our anniversary," she said, giving me a gentle smile.

I smiled back. "I'd rather be on a beach in Belize," I replied. "Maybe next year."

Katharina's presence was a calming one for me throughout my two weeks of treatment. She spent hours at my side, leaving only to spend the night in nearby rooms that she'd arranged through Airbnb or through a friend.

To lift her spirits and mine, she had also arranged for friends to visit her from Keene. Occasionally I would wake up to familiar faces at my bedside. I remember Jakob and Max, both of whom also spent hours at my side. Our friend Anna Guatieri stopped by and joked that I looked like I was getting plenty to eat.

"I was going to bring you some Greek food, but it looks like you don't need it," she said, giving me her usual mischievous smile.

"I'm not actually eating much," I answered. "It's mostly water weight. And if I could keep any food down, I'd much rather eat yours. I've had enough of hospital food for a lifetime."

Getting out of bed for my daily walks was more difficult during the second week. For one thing, there was no grace period before the side effects kicked in. They began with the first dose of the week, and I quickly settled into a routine of chills, shakes, itchiness, nausea, and diarrhea, punctuated by fitful slumber under the influence of Demerol. My bed's alarm had also been activated, which meant a nurse had to come in and disarm it every time I tried to leave the bed.

"I'm sorry about that, but it's for your own safety," Virginia Seery explained. "We've had too many patients fainting when they tried to go the bathroom during their second week of treatment."

Not wanting to keep Seery and the rest of the nursing staff from more important work, I decided to halt my walks. On the fourth day of treatment, a blood test revealed I had very low potassium levels, which meant I received an infusion of potassium instead of my normal dose. By Friday afternoon I decided, and Seery and Dr. McDermott agreed, that I had had enough after ten doses-- enough to call it a week.

They sent me home on Saturday. I weighed 195 pounds, but the nurse assured me that much of that was water weight.

"I wouldn't be surprised if you lost twenty pounds, especially after you take your Furosemide," she added.

She turned out to be right. A week later, I was down to 175, a weight I hadn't seen since my college days. My appetite was beginning to come back, but I still felt too weak to go back to work.

It would be another four weeks before I was scanned again to see whether the two weeks of treatment had had enough of an impact on my tumors to warrant another round. It seemed counterintuitive to hope for shrinkage, knowing that it would trigger the green light for another round of treatment. It may make me a glutton for punishment, but I was hoping for exactly that.

17 Not Enough Shrinkage

I returned to work two weeks after my last HDIL-2 treatment, regaining more of my mental and physical strength with each passing day. I had been out for five weeks in all—long enough to feel guilty about missing so much work, but also excited about getting caught up with colleagues and projects that had been put on hold during my time off.

The pace of life had picked up with the arrival of the freshmen class for Orientation Week. I quickly settled into my daily routine—waking up at 6:15 am, and out the door an hour later for the drive down to campus, which brought me to my office in Converse Hall by about 8:30. In the car, I made sure to urge on my immune system by listening to Gerald White's guided imagery exercises, visualizing cancer-conquering white blood cells stimulated by the treatment I had just endured.

College campuses in the fall are bustling places, with both professors and students eager (in theory, at least) to resume their teaching and learning, supported by staff who were working through the summer anyway. Amherst College was a place of beauty that autumn. The Holyoke mountain range shimmered with brilliant hues of red, orange, and yellow from the top of Memorial Hill, while in the late afternoon shafts of light from the setting sun shone golden rays onto the brick façade and white columns of Johnson Chapel.

Much less idyllic were my test results. One set of scans, taken a month after my treatment, showed that the numerous tumors in my lungs and lymph nodes, as well as the one near my spleen, had not yet been affected by the treatment. They hadn't grown, thankfully, but those few that had shrunk had done so only very slightly. Virginia Seery had told me by phone that I'd be re-scanned in another two months. Those scan results would provide more guidance as to whether it made sense for me to undergo another cycle of HDIL-2 treatment.

I thought about my upcoming scans occasionally, but mostly tried to focus on work—tasks such as planning and writing stories for the college's homepage and reaching out to media outlets with story pitches.

Many of these pitches focused on what I considered to be our best story: that Amherst College had evolved from being an *elitist* school to being an *elite* school. There were still plenty of Audis, BMWs and Mercedes in the student parking lots, but the percentage of students who were from low-income backgrounds, and who had therefore received generous financial aid packages, was among the highest in the nation.

(This was largely thanks to an endowment that, back then, was about $1.7 billion—a hefty sum for a college with a relatively small enrollment of only1,800 students. But it meant we could offer admission and financial aid packages made up of grants, not loans to the brightest and most talented students from around the world, regardless of their ability to pay.)

In early October, I headed into Boston for my scans, which I'd scheduled on a Saturday to avoid missing any more work than I already was. A few days later, Seery called to tell me the results.

"It looks like everything is stable, with slight shrinkage in a few spots," she said. It wasn't exactly what I had been hoping to hear; it looked like I hadn't been one of the lucky responders, that ten percent or so who showed dramatic enough shrinkage after the first two weeks of treatment to warrant proceeding with weeks three and four.

"So do I come in for another round of treatment?" I asked.

"I haven't discussed your results with Dr. Mier yet," she replied. "Why don't we talk about that when you come in next week for your appointment?"

So it was that Katharina and I found ourselves driving once more into Boston to find out what the next step would be in my treatment. Our first appointment at Beth Israel was with Dr. Erik Uhlmann, the neurologist who'd preserved my long weekend away with my family, to discuss the results of my recent brain MRI.

Dr. Uhlmann, a tall and angular gentleman with close-cropped hair, was a native of Hungary and spoke with a quiet, accented voice.

"The first thing to say is that is that MRI looks great," he said. "There's nothing new, and the spot we treated looks like it's healing nicely."

"That *is* good news," Katharina said, smiling at me.

"I still think you should come in again in two months for another MRI," Dr. Uhlmann added. "The plus side of the Cyberknife treatment is that there are very few side effects. But it's also very targeted. If there's anything else new happening in the brain, it doesn't get treated. And if this happened once, it can happen again—possibly not, but it can. The only way to know is to do the MRIs."

"Would there any big harm in coming in three months?" I asked. "I have some spots on my lungs, and I'm on a three-month scan cycle for those."

"You can certainly have it done every three months instead of every two months," he said. "It's more about a level of comfort. Say we find a new spot. I hope we don't, but suppose we do. Maybe it's ten millimeters instead of six millimeters. Then we would feel bad, because we could have done the MRI earlier."

"What's the probability of having more brain mets anyway, since I've had one already?" I asked. "Has that ever been studied?"

"Well, you know, everybody's different," he said. "It's hard to know. But if it happened once, it can happen again. It all depends. Sometimes it happens only once, but often there's more cancer cells in the blood and they settle somewhere in the brain, in a place where it's more comfortable for them, and they grow faster. Then a couple months later we see the new tumor, we zap it, and we're all good. Or maybe there are at least a couple cells in the blood all the time, and it keeps coming and coming. That's also possible.

"How about this?" he suggested. "We do a couple scans every two months, address the possibility there are cancer cells swirling around, and we catch them," he said. "But once we do that two times, then we go to every three months."

While I appreciated Dr. Uhlmann's conservative approach, I was worried about missing too much work for medical appointments. So we agreed that I would think about it and decide whether to schedule my MRI for two or three months hence.

"Let's see what Virginia and Dr. Mier think," I said to Katharina, as we headed to the hematology/oncology floor for our next appointment. "I can't imagine they'll think that one month will make a huge difference."

Indeed, that turned out to be the case. "I would recommend doing all the scans in three months," Dr. Mier said as we all settled into our seats in the examining room. "No one *likes* to drive into Boston to spend the whole day here. Let's wait until after the holidays and do all your scans in one day."

In addition to the brain MRI, I had also received CT scans of my chest, pelvis, and abdomen the previous week. Dr. Mier explained that overall, there was slight shrinkage in a few of my metastases, slight growth in a few others, and no change in a few more.

"It's not really enough information to guide a decision, except to say there's no major change in the overall amount of tumor you have," he said. "Sometimes we can get rid of the disease completely; that's always the selling point of interleukin-2. But in a lot more patients, you get this period of no progression that can be remarkably durable." His eyes brightened as he recalled a case from his past. "My personal record is actually eight years. I had a patient undergo HDIL-2; his tumors didn't really shrink, they just never grew afterwards. Which was fortunate for him, since we didn't really have any other drugs at the time.

"That's an extreme case, though," he acknowledged. "Eight years is quite long. What I would do is re-scan you in three months. As long as we keep tracking you, there are lots of other drugs we can try, including some that work through the immune system, that are extremely promising. Then there are other drugs based on other mechanisms of action that are out there. "But no one's saying they're curative. Immune therapies, on the other hand, present a possibility. There's one we're particularly optimistic about—it's currently investigational in nature—called PD-1."

I recalled hearing something about an ongoing trial for PD-1, and told him so.

He nodded. "We have a trial going, but it's filled," he said. "That's the way these things go; they start and they stop, then they start, then they stop again. Right now we don't have access to the one antibody we'd really want for you. Once the drug is FDA-approved, you won't have to fit the eligibility criteria for a clinical trial, but that may be some time off, so clinical trials are the only way to get access to it. It's not a reliable way to get access to a drug, but at certain points, it's the only way." He shrugged. "You certainly would be perfect candidate for it. Who knows? There may be trials that open up down the road."

I looked at Katharina, then at Virginia Seery, then back at Dr. Mier.

"So...watch and wait is what you're recommending?"

Dr. Mier nodded. "Unless your disease is taking over the body and you need urgent therapy, I think the best thing to do for now is simply to stand down. You still might get some delayed benefit from the HDIL-2. There are some tumors in your system that, for reasons that are unclear, *have* shrunk—not enough to warrant exposing you to those side effects for another cycle of HDIL-2, but certainly indicative that your immune system knows what it's doing."

I couldn't help feeling a boost of pride in my immune system. *I'm trying, goddammit. If my white blood cells hadn't killed off my tumors, they were at least keeping them from growing too fast.*

"If, on the other hand, the disease starts moving along, we would propose to put you on trial of an anti-PD-1 antibody, if we could access one," Dr. Mier continued. "If we can't get you on one of those, there are other drugs we can try, though none of them are potentially curative."

"When do you think these drugs will be available to everyone?" Katharina asked.

"It's hard to say, but I don't think it will be that long," the doctor replied. "There's too much competition. If you want the long and short of it, we started out with a little company called Medarex, who developed this drug for melanoma called ipi, or ipilimumab. They sold this drug to Bristol-Myers, and Bristol-Myers is now developing another PD-1 drug, as well.

"Now, because there's a hint that this might be an effective target, Merck—that's another large company—has an anti-PD1 drug, and there's even a little company called CureTech that's putting out an anti-PD1 drug, though theirs may or may not be as good."

I was very curious to hear more—about the science, not the business side of it—but I was also mindful that Dr. Mier and Seery had other patients to see, so I decided to hold my questions until later. *Maybe if and when they offer me a slot in a clinical trial.*

"So that's what I would like to do," Dr. Mier said, wrapping things up. "We'll scan after the holidays and see where we stand. If we don't have our backs up against the wall, and we're not really pressed, I'd rather just wait until PD-1 is available."

"That sounds good to me," I said, and we said our goodbyes and left.

As Katharina and I made our way back to Keene, I felt a sense of satisfaction and relief. True, my body hadn't responded quite as much as I had been hoping for. But I was encouraged that my immune system seemed to be working hard to keep my tumor growth in check.

Granted, it was hard to say whether the HDIL-2 was having a slight impact or whether other factors were at play, such as my regular use of guided imagery and my devotion to exercise and to meditation. Whatever it was, the order of the day would be "watch and wait" for the next three months, and for that I was grateful. My goal would be to live life as normally as possible.

What I had no way of knowing was that my professional life over the next few months would be the furthest thing possible from normal.

18 Working with Cancer

While it may seem difficult to believe, there *were* other things in my life at this time causing me headaches at least as bad as a Cyberknife treatment.

It started with a t-shirt—a deeply offensive t-shirt. A few days after my medical appointment in Boston, an Amherst student named Dana Bolger wrote a column in an online student magazine about a crude and distasteful t-shirt that members of an underground fraternity had designed, produced, and worn the previous spring.

"Do you wonder what sexism and misogyny look like in 2012?" Bolger wrote. "Imagine a drawing of a woman. She's clad only in a bra and a thong. She's got bruises on her side. There's an apple jammed in her mouth. And she's stretched out, tied up, suspended from a spit, and roasting over a fire."

"You don't have to imagine," Bolger continued. "Last April, a fraternity at Amherst designed this image, stuck it on a t-shirt, and sold the shirt to students in honor of the frat's annual pig-roast party. By the way, there *is* a pig depicted on the shirt. It's in the corner, smoking a cigar, and watching the woman roast. The words 'Roasting Fat Ones Since 1847' appear above the image."

In her article, Bolger took college administrators to task for not punishing the individual students involved in designing and printing the t-shirts, as well as for downplaying the issue of sexual assault on college campuses. The cartoonish image on the t-shirt, which the column had featured, was widely shared on Facebook

121

and Twitter, quickly becoming an embarrassingly apt symbol for the hateful attitudes that at least some of the male students at Amherst seemed to harbor toward women.

A few days after Dana Bolger's column was published, Amherst's new president wrote a letter to the campus community, officially condemning the t-shirt and affirming her commitment to examining and, if necessary, overhauling procedures for addressing incidents of sexual misconduct.

"The failure to respect the dignity, the boundaries, and the integrity of others violates the terms under which we are gathered as a community at this College," wrote Biddy Martin. "Indeed, it makes community impossible. And it will not be tolerated."

• • •

And for a while, that seemed to be the end of it. It wasn't until a week later, as I was resting at home, stretched out on a couch with my laptop on my chest, checking in on Amherst's Facebook and Twitter accounts, that I noticed Amherst College popping up in tweets and Facebook posts an awful lot—and not in a good way.

"This needs more attention," one tweet said. "How Amherst College ignores rapists and mistreats survivors. How many others are like this?"

"Just wow," read another post. "So much strength so much courage for dealing with the shittiest administration ever."

I clicked a link included in many of the posts, and was connected to a guest column in the college's independent student newspaper, *The Amherst Student*. Written by a former student named Angie Epifano, the 5000-word article was titled "An Account of Sexual Assault at Amherst College."

"When you're being raped, time does not stop," the article began. "Time does not speed up and jump ahead like it does when you are with friends. Instead, time becomes your nemesis; it slows to such an excruciating pace that every second becomes an hour, every minute a year, and the rape becomes a lifetime.

"On May 25, 2011, I was raped by an acquaintance in Crossett Dormitory.

Some nights, I can still hear the sounds of his roommates on the other side of the door, unknowingly talking and joking as I was held down."

Epifano recounted how she felt compelled to go public with her story because she was so disillusioned with how she was treated. As I read Epifano's account of her interactions with college administrators and counselors when she reported the rape about a year later, I found myself dismayed and disappointed by what she described. Among many other accusations, she wrote that Amherst administrators "cover up survivors' stories, cook their books to discount rapes, pretend that withdrawals never occur, quell attempts at change, and sweep sexual assaults under a rug."

Epifano wrote that she went to the college's counseling center, "as they always tell you to do, and spoke about how genuinely sad I was at Amherst, how much I wanted to leave, and how scared I was on a daily basis." When she mentioned considering suicide as a way to deal with her depression, campus police were notified, and she was driven to Cooley Dickinson Hospital, where she was admitted into the psychiatric ward.

Epifano described the four days she spent there, being released only after she dug in her heels and refused to give in to the college's demand that a parent monitor her from a nearby hotel for two weeks to ensure she was capable of returning to campus.

As a result of this, Epifano was denied an opportunity to study abroad in South Africa, citing administrators' concerns about her mental health. She eventually decided to withdraw from the college and work on urging changes in how sexual assaults are investigated and resolved.

"At one point, I hated Amherst with an indescribable amount of fury, but I do not hate the school anymore," she wrote toward the end of her essay. "Amherst took a lot from me, but they gave me some of the greatest gifts imaginable: self-confidence, my closest friends, intellectual curiosity, and endless personal strength. For these things, I am forever grateful. For everything else, I stand back and behold the college with a feeling of melancholia."

• • •

After I'd finished reading her essay, a few things became clear.

As the college's director of public affairs, one of my chief responsibilities was to safeguard the reputation of Amherst College. However, as a former reporter who had covered higher education in Illinois, I had learned that universities were powerful institutions and that the administrators who worked there were only too capable of misdeeds, cover-ups, and astonishing lapses in judgment.

I knew it was only a matter of hours before the media would be calling, asking for a response to these horrendous allegations. As a college, we needed to respond compassionately, transparently, and promptly, while also devoting ourselves to investigating what had happened, correcting our mistakes and committing ourselves to doing better in the future.

I said just that in an email I wrote that evening, addressed to President Biddy Martin and other senior administrators. I also suggested we meet the next morning to prepare a response to this potentially fast-moving crisis.

In public, Biddy had perfected her role as a matronly, avuncular authority figure, but she hadn't risen from being an assistant professor in German studies and women's studies at Cornell to president at Amherst by being a passive pushover. As Don Randel, the former president of the University of Chicago and her immediate predecessor at Cornell, put it: "Biddy has a disarming smile, a ready laugh, and a sense of humor that she does not exercise at the expense of others. But there is no mistaking that she is tough-minded when the occasion demands it."

On this morning, the occasion certainly demanded it, and Martin was not smiling. Rather, she was furious and seemingly disgusted with the allegations that Epifano had made in her article. At a round table in her office, surrounded by her senior staff, she argued forcefully that Epifano's story should be acknowledged for what it was: a horrifying, tragic account of a young woman being very poorly served by the very system that was supposed to protect her.

I agreed and said we should respond quickly, not by taking issue with Epifano's allegations but by pledging to investigate them and changing our policy as necessary to ensure the health and safety of our students going forward.

"I think the key is to be as transparent as possible," I said. "The worst thing we could do is to go into a defensive crouch and say 'no comment.' We need to commit to investigating this and to doing everything in our power to make sure something like this doesn't happen again."

"I agree," Martin said. "I want a statement on the homepage by noon that articulates how horrified I am by all of this, and I want you to begin writing it."

After getting some initial thoughts from Martin, I shut my laptop, tucked it under my arm, and returned to my office to begin working on the statement. As I shut the door behind me, I exchanged a quick glance with my boss, Susan, who would fill me in on how the rest of the meeting went later in the day.

Martin's response was posted to the College's website by early afternoon, less than 24 hours after Epifano's letter first appeared. In it, she acknowledged that Epifano's account of her sexual assault and its aftermath was "horrifying" and that the college's response to it left much to be desired.

"Clearly the administration's responses to reports have left survivors feeling that they were badly served—that must change, and change immediately," she wrote, and announced the college was launching an internal investigation into Epifano's account of her sexual assault and its unfortunate aftermath.

Martin vowed to take other steps as well, such as forming a Special Oversight Committee on Sexual Misconduct, overhauling the college's Counseling Center, and bringing in clinicians from Harvard University's McLean Center to provide counseling and policy advice to students and staff.

She directed me to work with colleagues around campus to develop and launch a "Sexual Respect" website which, among other things, would explain students' options for reporting sexual misconduct and outline steps the college had already taken to address sexual violence.

But if anyone at the college thought this meant an end to negative media attention, they were sorely mistaken. In early November, an online publication called the *Good Men Project* published the suicide note that former Amherst student Trey Malone left behind before jumping to his death off the Sunshine Skyway Bridge in Tampa Bay. Malone wrote that he was committing suicide in part because of the way college staff treated him after he reported being sexually assaulted. Like Epifano, Malone had less-than-positive reviews of his treatment by administrators.

"What began as an earnest effort to help on the part of Amherst, became an emotionless hand washing," he said in his final note. "In those places I should've received help, I saw none."

Malone's suicide note spread like wildfire through social media, adding to the chorus of criticism toward the college. It, combined with Dana Bolger's article and Epifano's column, created a public relations crisis unlike anything Amherst had ever seen.

I spent hours working with colleagues, editors, and reporters, arranging interviews, updating the college's sexual respect website, and making sure that our response and our commitment to changing our policy was communicated to the outside world. This was no easy task; conveying both a willingness to reform and action steps taken is a difficult narrative to convey, not least of which is because it does not easily reduce to soundbites. Federal legislation called Title IX obligates colleges and universities to investigate and rule on all cases of reported sexual assault, even those in which there is little or no physical evidence. Prosecutors have been reluctant to take on cases which rely solely on witness testimony, finding them difficult to prove beyond a reasonable doubt to juries. Colleges like Amherst are still required to review and try to make sense of these often murky cases, the vast majority of which involve consumption of alcohol and conflicting statements. Now, Amherst was being loudly accused of setting up a disciplinary system that favored perpetrators rather than victims of sexual assault. Enforcement of Title IX fell to the Department of Justice's Office of Civil Rights, and though a complaint hadn't yet been filed against the College, it seemed only a matter of time before one was. It made good moral sense—as well as good legal sense—to demonstrate our commitment to being held accountable for our shortcomings, backed up with forceful action.

Meanwhile, students at other colleges were coming forward with similar stories. These played a huge role in pushing colleges and universities across the nation to analyze and revamp their policies and procedures surrounding sexual assault on college campuses in an effort to ensure that victims' interests were given at least as much credence as the rights of the accused.

With so much going on at work, the months slipped by almost unnoticed. Though it seems impossible to believe, I had forgotten about my illness—first for hours, then for days at a time. I had learned a few things about coping with stress, though, and was diligent about exercising regularly. I also remained committed to meditation, guided imagery, and good nutrition.

But as 2013 was ushered in, I saw the calendar begin to fill up with appointments. CT scans, a brain MRI, and a follow-up appointment with Dr. Mier and Dr. Uhlmann were all right around the corner.

I was soon to find out whether my immune system was holding its own against the cancer within me.

19 Watching and Waiting

On a cold January morning, I found myself driving into Boston for my latest round of scans. The waiting room was like a crowded deli counter, with patients taking numbers and waiting until theirs was called. I filled out my intake form, making sure to point out in writing that I was missing a kidney and that my dose of contrast dye should thus be adjusted.

I settled into an armchair, and the radiology technician tightened a strip of rubber around my upper arm, just above the elbow. He lightly slapped my forearm before smoothly poking a needle into a vein and inserting my IV line. He taped it up and capped off the clear rubber tube before leading me to the room where the donut-shaped CT scan machine awaited—the first stop in a day packed with appointments, which included a brain MRI, a bone scan, and me guzzling water on the drive home to flush the dye out of my kidney as soon as possible.

A few days later, I sent an email to Dr. Mier because I hadn't heard anything from him. I didn't want to appear too anxious, so instead of asking for the results directly, my first email congratulated him for a research grant he had secured that I had read about in a news release on the web. I hoped he would get the hint.

In short order, a reply from Dr. Mier was in my inbox:

"Thanks, we're excited about this award since there were only two funded out of forty-four applications. BTW—I saw your bone scan—it doesn't show anything particularly alarming. We'll see you next week."

Okay, so my bones are fine, I thought. *What about my brain, lungs and lymph nodes?*

So I sent another email:

"Great news; did you happen to see the other scans?"

As the days ticked past with no answer, worst case scenarios—blossoming tumors, debilitating treatment, severe fatigue, hand sores, foot and throat sores—all burrowed themselves into my consciousness. I tried to keep these worries at bay with deep breaths, more iPod sessions with Gerald White and Jon Kabat-Zinn, and the occasional tablet of lorazepam. I even added a new mantra to my mental playlist: *Don't assume the worst will happen.*

Three *very* long days later, Dr. Mier sent his response:

"The head scan shows only the residual abnormality from the previously treated metastasis—no growth or new disease. The body CT shows minimal growth of some lymph nodes in the chest—not enough to warrant any action at the present time."

It was news I could live with. It wasn't the worst-case scenario, but it wasn't encouraging news, either. Statistically speaking, I was in the broad middle of outcomes. I hadn't been cured, but my disease wasn't racing ahead aggressively, either.

The next week I drove into Boston for two more appointments—the first with Dr. Erik Uhlmann, the Hungarian-born neurologist who was tracking my brain, and the next with Dr. Mier, who I hoped to quiz about my chances of scoring a ticket for a clinical trial "rock concert."

After greeting Katharina and me, Dr. Uhlmann administered a quick sequence of tests to determine my brain function—asking me to track his fingers with my eyes, touch my nose with my index finger, and to walk heel-to-toe "like you're on a high wire."

"You function," Katharina joked as I breezed through the tasks.

"Now let's review your medication list," Dr. Uhlmann said. "Any change there?"

I leaned my head over to read through the list on his screen's display.

"I'm not taking the Lovastatin anymore," I pointed out. "I think I've got bigger fish to fry than borderline high cholesterol."

Dr. Uhlmann smiled slightly and continued scrolling down the list.

"Do you need any prescriptions filled?"

"Well, the lorazepam that you gave me last time is just about done."

"What do you take it for?" he asked.

"Just general de-stressing at night," I said.

"Fine," he said, making a note to renew the prescription.

"I'm also taking Xgeva to help keep bone mets at bay, and curcumin; I've read that it might do something," I added.

I had discovered online that curcumin, a spice common in many Asian and Indian dishes, has potentially powerful tumor-fighting properties, in addition to being a strong antioxidant that can help prevent or delay damage to healthy cells. The articles ranged in tone from whimsical ("curcumin and cancer cells: how many ways can curry kill tumor cells selectively?") to quite technical. One experiment, described in the journal *Brain Research* (performed in test tubes, not patients), found that curcumin both prevented brain tumor formation and killed brain tumor cells. Another, published in *Nutrition and Cancer*, found curcumin makes tumors more sensitive to chemotherapy and radiation, potentially enhancing these forms of cancer treatment.

That said, there's some debate about how exactly curcumin gets absorbed. The type I was taking was infused with pepper extract, which supposedly helps the body absorb it better. But unfortunately, most medical researchers don't do many studies on natural medications, which is why the information was scarce and conflicting. Still, I felt it was worth a try.

Coming to the end of my medications list, I paused before asking a question I'd been curious about for a while, but always felt too foolish to ask a medical researcher about. "What about visualization? As a neurologist, you might know how the brain works in this area; can I use the power of the mind to focus my immune system on fighting cancer? Or is that total hocus-pocus?"

"Probably not," Dr. Uhlmann said carefully. "We don't know exactly how these things work, and I'm not an expert in these things. What I can tell you, though, is that placebos *do* work. We don't know exactly how, but if you give somebody a placebo, a sugar pill, it works for a number of cases."

Dr. Uhlmann's dark eyes, embedded in his lean, angular face, looked first at me, and then Katharina. "Now, you know that doctors don't just give out placebos to people unless they're part of a clinical trial, and it's for research purposes. And you might ask, 'If it works so often, why don't we?' The truth is, we just don't think it's ethical. We would have to lie to you for the placebo effect to work, telling you the pill contains medicine that will help you, when it really has nothing of the sort.

"It's a dilemma for us, but there *are* a number of things that placebos help with, and visualization is kind of like that. I would imagine that something is going on there that we don't yet understand. One day, maybe we will know and it will be used for healing.

"At the same time," he added, "I'm a scientist, so I want to do things that I know work. I don't want to give you things that are not proven. So we have to find a kind of balance between promising things and trying different things while also doing the things that we know are proven."

I remembered Gerald White's strong belief that traditional medicine should be harnessing the placebo effect's power on a massive scale. Yet Dr. Uhlmann's cogent explanation of why handing out placebo pills would be unethical made sense, too. Regardless, the appointment moved on to the matter at hand—what the radiologist had seen in the MRI from the week before. The issues I was most concerned with were whether the small scar which showed on my cerebellum represented normal healing, and whether having been treated for a brain tumor would disqualify me for any clinical trials.

Dr. Uhlmann said the scar was perfectly normal and no cause for alarm. "The Cyberknife leaves a spot like that because it's very powerful; it's like a laser beam. But it doesn't disqualify you for anything. Most trials would exclude active brain tumors, but this one is not active. This is treated and stable. Every trial is different, but most trials would be okay with this."

That was music to my ears, and Katharina and I headed off to our appointment with Dr. Mier in good spirits.

• • •

I always looked forward to seeing Virginia Seery, the nurse for the hematology and oncology unit at Beth Israel. Ever since my two hospitalizations for HDIL-2 treatment, Seery had been the person most involved in my care, and was always willing to spend the time explaining my treatment options and answering questions about my cancer.

She started things off this time by inquiring how I'd been.

Let's stick to the basics here, I thought. *No need for a long monologue.*

"In general, pretty good," I said. "The last three months, I haven't been thinking about cancer too much. I've been working, enjoying the snow. We've been skiing quite a bit—downhill and cross-country."

An enthusiastic conversation about skiing followed. I had learned to ski as a young adult in a study abroad program by serving as a guinea pig. Teachers in Austria were often asked to take students on week-long ski trips, and flatlanders like me were paired with student teachers. It worked out great for me, and sparked a lifelong hobby.

Seery smiled as we discussed our shared interest, then tactfully steered the conversation to health, summarizing the scan results and how they might influence treatment options.

"The CT scan *does* show a few lymph nodes that are a little bit bigger," she said. "Dr. Mier and I were just talking, and I was asking him what his opinion was."

"What did he think?" I replied.

"Well, there are two schools of thought," she began. "One is that you could start treatment right now. The other is that you could wait. You're feeling good, you're not thinking about cancer that much, and we can watch you closely. TKI medicines like Sutent all carry the risk of side effects, so we'd like to make sure we start you on any new medication for a reason, as opposed to just a little change on a scan.

"If you would be comfortable sitting tight for the next three months, Dr. Mier would favor that. We're still thinking about a PD-1 anti-body trial, one that combines a TKI with this new immunotherapy. We'd rather go that route, and if we give you a TKI now, you won't be eligible for that trial. This is the game we play—seeing what's coming down the pike and keeping our options open. It's a little nerve-wracking, because we never know when a slot can open up, but we'll try to keep you in the loop as far as what's happening."

I had my own reasons for wanting to avoid TKI treatment. I had this notion that exercise boosted the immune system, and TKIs would make it hard to exercise, so I hoped to avoid these targeted therapies for as long as possible. I didn't want to give up my active lifestyle. Rational or not, I didn't see myself being able to do that if went on Sutent or similar drugs.

"Are there any trials that are PD-1 exclusively?" I asked.

"There's nothing open right now," she replied. "If there was an opening, we could put you on it. Which is progress in itself; the last time we saw you, I don't think we would have been eligible."

"I'd prefer that," I said. "The straight-up PD-1."

At that point, there was a light knock-knock on the door and Dr. Mier poked his head into the room.

I had really come to like Dr. Mier; he always offered a smile as he greeted me, and that smile always gave me hope, conveying both optimism and empathy—even if he sometimes had to deliver grim news. "I gather you went over the PD-1 stuff?" he said as he settled into a chair.

I nodded.

"Right now, the only way you can get these drugs is by being on a clinical trial," he said. "There are a half dozen or more trials being planned now that four companies are working in this area. But a trial that combines a PD-1 agent with a TKI is the one that's actually imminent."

Dr. Mier gave me an encouraging smile. "Now, your scan doesn't mandate an urgent need to do anything," he said. "In the brain, we didn't see any new spots; you may be done with that for good.

"On the bone scans," he continued, "the radiologists are kind of waffling on whether there's anything there. They can't tell if there's a very low activity tumor or whether it's just where the tendon goes into the bone. On the CT scan of the rest of your body, you've got one lymph node that's grown a little bit, but everything else is rock stable."

"So would you say it's relatively good news?" I asked.

"I wouldn't feel the need to qualify it," Dr. Mier said. "I'd say it's very good news. That one lymph node *has* gotten a bit bigger, but in the grand scheme of things, with everything else that you have, I would say it's a very good report. It does not indicate an urgent need to be stampeded into anything. Until there's a protocol that we find to be particularly attractive, I'm willing to simply do nothing at all and scan in three months.

"You're not that atypical, by the way," he added. "Maybe it's the effect of the HDIL-2, but there's a sizable fraction of patients whose disease progresses in a sort of geologic time frame, one that doesn't mandate urgent intervention on the part of the physician.

"I would still like you take advantage of PD-1 at some point," he assured me. "That's by far the most exciting thing in the field right now. Some of them you won't be qualified for, and some you might turn your nose up at because they have multiple agents, including TKIs, so unless you have your back up against the wall, I would hold out for the PD-1s, either in a trial or after FDA approval."

Now came the part of my appointment where I could ask all the little questions I'd jotted down in the past few months. I was mindful of Dr. Mier's limited time, but I felt it was important for me to probe other treatment options.

"About my lung and lymph node lesions," I asked. "Can they be surgically addressed?"

"Probably not," he replied. "They're in a high traffic area. One of yours is right at the carina, which is the bifurcation of the windpipe, where it splits into left and right. Nerves go through there, it's right behind the heart...it's hard to get to, from a technical standpoint. That's not to say it *can't* be done, but we'd typically only do that if the area itself needed to be cleared; if it was inhibiting your normal functions."

"So when do the tumors get to a size where treatment becomes necessary?"

"It isn't so much size as what they're doing to nearby structures," he corrected. "A strategically located lymph node can occlude or obstruct the bronchus, and it doesn't have to be very big to do so. Of course, the minute we see something that suggests they're interfering with the flow of air into certain regions of lung, we start to consider options like the Cyberknife. That's actually one of the dominant uses for it."

We discussed a number of other hypothetical treatment options, including one particularly interesting option called photodynamic therapy, which drastically increases the body's sensitivity to light to better kill off tumors. But in the end, Dr. Mier's recommendation didn't change. "For you, right now, I think the best plan would be to wait for the right PD-1 trial."

"Alright, then. I guess we'll just wait and see," I said, and then congratulated him again on his recent research grant. After years of interviewing professors, I knew how much they enjoyed discussing their work, and how infrequently many of them were asked about it.

"It sounds interesting," I said. "Is there anything there to get excited about?"

In addition to seeing patients, Dr. Mier directs the Biologics Therapy lab research program at Beth Israel and is an associate professor of medicine at Harvard Medical School. He quickly warmed to his subject. "The study has to do primarily with trying to sustain the effects of the TKI drugs, like Sutent and Votrient," he explained. "Tumors can find their way around those drugs easily; it takes very little time for a tumor to figure out a way around TKIs. When that happens, there's a tumor suppressor gene that gets clipped off, and that used to be the limitation of TKIs.

"Now we have drugs that restore these genes' functions, called HDM2 antagonists. Use those alongside TKIs like Sutent, and you get a sustained anti-tumor effect. They basically deny the cancer cells an escape from the TKIs. Remember, TKI drugs work by targeting the blood vessels that feed the tumors, slowly starving off the cancer. Problem is that 'slowly' part. The tumors experience progressive starvation, and that triggers all sorts of adaptations. *That's* what the HDM2 antagonists are meant to nullify.

"Now, the purpose of our research is to try to figure out why these work well together. The HDM2 antagonists we're working with are barely in Phase 1 testing, but we still hope to have kidney cancer studies in testing within a year or two. Right now, we're basically restricted to using mice."

It all sounded so promising, and yet *just* out of reach.

But all that could change with time. Playing the watch and wait game could be nerve-wracking, but I'd become better at putting the cancer out of my mind. Even from my perspective, waiting things out seemed to be the best option.

Katharina and I stood up together and thanked Dr. Mier and Seery.

"Good luck with all your other patients," I said, "and we'll see you in the spring."

Katharina and I headed back home, driving through the cold, dark late afternoon. It looked like we had three more months of sitting on our hands.

Maybe a trip someplace warm would help keep things stable.

20 Hawaiian Healing

While we gamely skied our cross country loops through an especially punishing series of snowstorms and weeks of frigid temperatures, by the end of January, Katharina and I were both ready for an escape from winter.

We considered visiting Belize again, but chose Hawaii somewhat impulsively after watching *Violent Hawaii*—which was not, as it sounds, a *Hawaii Five-O* knockoff, but a nature documentary exploring the volcanic fury, raging mountaintop blizzards, dangerous rock-slides, monster waves, and even tsunamis that visited the state.

Not that we were hoping to encounter any of these calamities, mind you. But it sure made the islands sound intriguing and full of adventure. After some online research, we picked Kauai. It appeared to be the least developed of the major islands, meaning the mega-resorts were confined to two ends of the island, and offered plenty of access to coral reefs for snorkeling and national parks for hiking.

Based on the recommendation of my sister Anna in Chicago, we booked our reservations through Airbnb, at a location called "the Treehouse," and this time the connections worked to perfection. Katharina booked tickets for both of us: a direct flight from Boston to Los Angeles, then a brief layover, then a jet from LA to Lihue, where we rented a car and made our way to the Treehouse in Anahola, soaking up the moist, warm air, enjoying the glimpses of ocean and cresting waves, and laughing at the wild chickens we saw darting about the yards everywhere.

Our directions led us to the end of a dirt road just as it was getting dark. As we got out of the mid-sized Sentra, our motion triggered the outdoor lighting, illuminating a stairway leading to the main entrance and our host for the time being.

Ventura had fallen in love with Kauai during childhood trips there and was a top-notch innkeeper (if her overwhelmingly positive reviews online were any indication). Though not technically a treehouse, everything else at the Treehouse lived up to its billing. The property was nestled among several banana, coconut, palm, and papaya trees. Our room was snug but comfortable, and we slept well every night we were there.

That first morning, sipping coffee on the second-floor patio, we noticed the jagged green peaks of Kalalea Mountain looming in the distance. Ventura joined us on the patio and told us that the mountain, as well as the village of Anahola, had great importance in Hawaiian history and culture.

"There's a sacred birthing temple that goes back thousands of years at the base of the mountain," she said. "It's still guarded today by a Hawaiian priest."

We were still planning our day, wondering whether it made sense to hit the ocean right away or plan a hike first. It being winter, the waves were high, and Ventura advised against surfing lessons. Even snorkeling would be a challenge, according to our host, and it was important not to underestimate the current and the force of the waves. The hikes we were considering could be dangerous, too, with plenty of cliffs, narrow ridges, and steep drop-offs.

Nancy did have some more positive recommendations. "When the Dalai Lama came to the Hawaiian Islands in 1994, he only asked to see two places, and both were on Kauai," she said. "Instead of asking to see the Na Pali Coast, he wanted to see Anahola and Polihale. When his hosts asked why, he said, 'We know Anahola is a portal where the souls or spirits enter this world and Polihale is where the souls or spirits exit this world.'"

At Ventura's suggestion, we connected with her friend Danny Hashimoto, a photographer, naturalist, and Kauai native who took us on a hike along a mostly unmarked trail on the Kalapa

Ridge, treating us to mountainous terrain thousands of feet above Waimea Canyon with stunning views of the Na Pali coastline far below. It wasn't the sacred location the Dalai Lama had visited, but it certainly was spectacular, with stomach clenching ridges that yielded spectacular vistas, with waves crashing so far below that they resembled a thin white line undulating on a massive canvas of deep blue.

Another day, taking off on our own, we hiked a stretch of the famous Na Pali coast, marveling at the lushness and misty beauty of a landscape that seemed too dramatic to be real. I plunged into a frigid pool fed by a waterfall that tumbled from a mountain that was shrouded in mist on one of the wettest spots on the planet. The water was bracing, but I stayed in until my body adjusted to its cool temperature.

Keeping Ventura's advice in mind, we avoided surfing beaches and headed instead for the beaches with coral reefs, which broke up the large waves before they hit shore. The surf still jostled us as we swam in the water, though, and it took a lot of strength to swim against the waves and hold our place above the reefs.

We also took a chance on snorkeling, using equipment that Ventura made available to her guests. We watched sea turtles and vibrant-hued fish like triggerfish, yellow tang, and stripers go about their lives in relative calm beneath the agitated surface water, oblivious to us watching them and the waves that rolled above them.

It was during one of these snorkeling sessions that I lost my wedding ring. I noticed it missing a few hours after we returned, as we settled down in our bed, exhausted yet satisfied after another day spent exploring the island.

I had managed to hold onto that ring through more than twenty-six years of marriage. I was sad, but I wasn't devastated. Yes, the ocean had claimed my ring. But now I had a reason to return to Kauai in the years ahead. Another reason to keep going year after year.

I've got to keep looking for my ring.

PART III

Taming the Beast

21 Playing the Clinical Trial Game

More than two years had passed since my original Stage IV cancer diagnosis. Despite the relative stability of my various tumors, I still worried about their slow growth even as I pictured my T cells munching on them. When I had the time for visualization exercises, that is. I was still working full time, but was feeling increasingly drained with each week that went by.

Katharina and I made this clear to Virginia Seery at our next appointment, which took place about a month after our trip to Hawaii and a few days after my latest scans.

"But generally you're feeling well?" Seery asked at the beginning of our appointment. "Have you noticed any wheezing? Shortness of breath?"

"Well, I'm still running and swimming," I replied. "At times when I inhale, I notice a wheeze, but I can work it out so it's not a consistent wheeze."

"If you can work it out, then it's probably not cancer related. How's your energy?"

"I would say my energy is okay, but I don't think it's great. When I come home from work, I'm pretty tired."

Katharina agreed. "It used to be I couldn't keep up with Peter; I lived with that all my life. But now we're about the same. Which isn't bad either," she said with a small smile. "Now I don't have to chase after him."

Seery nodded and smiled. "And how's work going?"

"Well, I want to work as long as I can, but I don't want to work myself into the ground either," I explained. "Jakob has two more years of college left, so it would be nice to work if I can." I shot her a knowing look and added, "Tuition isn't cheap."

"For sure," Seery said, and summarized my situation, as she saw it: "So for now, you're good with working, but you're thinking about options."

I nodded. "That's right. Sometimes it seems like there's too much to deal with. And I don't see it getting any easier. Someone in my office is going on maternity leave right when the fall semester starts. I'm happy for her, but it means I'll be doing some of her tasks, too. I don't think a bigger workload will be good, especially if I'm on treatment."

"Well, Dr. Mier and still I think you should hold out for the immune therapies," Seery said. "His take on it is that we do need *some* treatment, but we don't need it urgently."

At that moment, Dr. Mier himself appeared, and after a quick greeting, noted that my scans looked similar to three months earlier, with one exception. A tumor in my sub-carinal lymph node, located to the right of my esophagus, had grown since January. It now measured 3.7 by 2.1 centimeters, compared to 3 by 1.4 centimeters three months earlier.

"It's a little bit bigger than it was, but not alarmingly so," he said. "And you don't have anything else that's alarming. We worry most about this disease in vital organs like the brain, so we're much relieved that's not an issue."

From over his glasses he glanced at me and then Katharina, offering a reassuring smile. "So there isn't any rush to do anything," he said, echoing Seery's earlier statement. "We're still going to want to consider putting you on the list for these immune therapies that we discussed the last time you were here."

I'd spent the time since my last appointment researching immunotherapy drugs online, and though early clinical trial results looked promising in other types of cancers, I couldn't find anything about the response rates that kidney patients were showing from the immunotherapy trials.

"I don't know how many people have it go away completely, but a lot of people have major responses," Dr. Mier replied when I asked him about this. "The disease shrinks way down, but you'll still have this remnant that persists and continues to show up in scans. They're called spider clots, and it's difficult to say whether there's any active disease there."

Dr. Mier also explained that PD-1 was having another interesting effect on some patients in trials—it was causing their tumors to actually *swell* for a few months before shrinking.

"'Pseudo-progression' is the new term for this condition," Dr. Mier said. "We're now aware of this, and thankfully clinical trials don't demand an immediate result. So you're allowed to have people get worse on the first scan. But the bottom line is that well over half of patients are seeing their tumor load go below their initial baseline—in some cases down to twenty or thirty percent of what they had before."

"And these cancer cells don't develop a workaround that lets them come back?"

"We haven't seen that," Dr. Mier confirmed. "I'm not really sure why that is, but it's a fundamental distinction between immune-based and TKI-based treatments. Sutent kind of creates its own problems because it lowers the oxygen in the tumors, which granted is how the tumor is killed, but the areas that *aren't* killed are challenged by that hypoxia, and that actually makes some cancer cells grow more aggressively. The tumor cells change their metabolism so they need less oxygen, which allows them to grow faster. But the immune-based therapies don't do any of these things."

"And what about someone like me, who's had tumors spread to the brain and to bones—are the PD-1 drugs effective for that, too?" I asked.

"As far as I know, the immune system doesn't care," Dr. Mier answered. "We used to say that the immune system never works in the brain because IL-2 never works in the brain. But now we're back-pedaling."

"So now you think that the PD-1 drug *is* crossing the blood-brain barrier?"

"We *know* it is," he affirmed. "Both of the new checkpoint inhibitors work by releasing the immune system to work in the brain to a degree that IL-2 never did. We've been forced to admit that the dogma is wrong."

This all sounded pretty good to me, but Dr. Mier seemed a little less enthusiastic. "It's an exciting time, but I still think we should avoid jumping at whatever trial is available. Better to wait a bit, to see what unfolds," he said. "These are going to be investigational agents for the foreseeable future, so you'll have to get it through joining a formal trial."

A quick word on the process of drug approval: Drugs need to clear three phases of tests, each involving more patients, before they are reviewed for approval by the Food and Drug Administration. It's a process that can take years and billions of dollars of investment, and the possibility of failure exists at each step of the way if a drug doesn't significantly improve upon outcomes existing drugs already offer.

That's the theory, at least. In reality, many drugs seem to offer only incremental improvement over their predecessors to patients, but because they provide lucrative revenue streams for drug makers, they hit the market with relatively little issue.

I decided to test the waters on that front. "Are you as excited about the drugs that are close to getting approved as the ones that are at the beginning of the pipeline?" I asked.

"I'd say I'm more ambivalent," he replied after a moment's thought. "The best drug right now—on paper, at least—is a Merck compound aimed at the same protein, but it's not as far along in its development; it's still a Phase 1 drug. Meanwhile, the Bristol-Myers Squibb antibody has been in clinical testing for about four years now, so there's a huge amount of data regarding side effects and what the dose and schedule should be.

"It's all a bit of a game. People are acting as if the FDA's already signed off on the BMS drug, and now they're proposing combinations. There are a number of combination trials for both kidney cancer and melanoma patients planned for the months ahead, ones which combine the BMS drug with other treatments, including TKIs like Sutent."

"Even though they think the PD-1 on its own would be effective?"

"They think combining the two could be more effective," Dr. Mier said with a shrug.

Those TKIs again. It seemed like I just couldn't get away from them. *Better to be informed, then.*

"Let's say you get me on a trial with Sutent or Votrient and the PD-1," I began, "and it turns out that the side effects from the TKIs are quite high. When do we get to the point where you take me off the TKI and I continue on the PD-1 alone?"

Seery smiled. "He's smart," she said, looking at Dr. Mier.

"We just did that with a patient," he said with a grin. "You *do* have to be on the TKIs for at least a month to stay on the trial, but I don't see that being a problem with you. The usual problem we run into with clinical trial candidates is high blood pressure—we're talking 160 over 100, and that's while taking blood pressure medication. That's just not adequate. A lot of the TKI combination studies demand a blood pressure of 140 over 90 or less before you can be considered a candidate.

"And even if we're able to lower their blood pressure by increasing their medication, all that happens is they get put on Sutent and the PD-1 antibody and they immediately get in trouble with higher blood pressure or some other side effect associated with the TKIs, and they're off the trial. But as I've said, that won't be an issue for you.

"The requirement for one of the trials going now is that you have to receive half of the prescribed TKI cycle; otherwise, you're not allowed to continue at all. But if you get through that, and it's deemed in your interest to stop the TKI, you can stop it and continue the PD-1. Believe me; we're *very* aware of that option."

Katharina had been quietly absorbing this information and chimed in with a good question. "Is there any proof that the combination works better?"

"None yet, but this trial should provide that proof—we hope," he said. "And we're trying other combinations, too."

"Well, I'm willing to take the TKIs if it gives me access to the PD-1," I said. "I went through HDIL-2, and that was pretty rough stuff."

"If you can do that, you can do anything," Dr. Mier replied, and I couldn't help chuckling.

"No, really, I'm not joking," he insisted. "If HDIL-2 is a ten, this would be maybe a four or five. PD1 alone is a two as near as I can tell."

Dr. Mier looked at both of us. "So should we put you on the list?"

I looked at Katharina, who looked back. We didn't have to exchange words. We both knew we had little to lose.

"Please do," I said. "And thanks for the offer."

Alright, then. Let's take the plunge.

22 Informed Consent

July 2, 2013. Today was the day I would start backing my cancer into a corner where it could be ambushed by my T cells and reduced to a smoking glob of lifeless protoplasm.

At least, that was my sincere hope as I drove into Boston with Katharina to sign the forms indicating my consent to participate in a Phase 1 clinical trial being held at Beth Israel Deaconess Medical Center. The study's aim was to determine whether combining ipilimumab with the investigational antibody nivolumab lent the treatment a bigger impact and, if so, to discover the optimal dose. At the time, nivo was already in Phase 3 testing for other types of cancer such as melanoma, while ipi had been FDA-approved in the US for treatment of melanoma, under the brand name Yervoy.

Half the participants in this arm of the trial would receive a large dose of ipi, while the other half would receive a much smaller one (everyone would receive the same dose of nivo). The drugs would be delivered via an infusion every two weeks; the nivo–ipi portion of the trial would last three months, after which participants would switch to nivo only, with no end date listed, at least on the consent form.

The consent form also mentioned two other arms of the study, one which was combining nivo with Sutent, and another that combined nivo with Votrient, both meant to see whether targeted therapies that blocked the blood supply for tumors would work even better in combination with immune therapy.

149

Signing the form didn't technically mean I was in the trial, though. There was one more hurdle to clear before those crushed velvet ropes lifted for me, and it had to do with the small brain tumor that had been treated the previous year.

The trial monitors representing Bristol-Myers Squibb needed to be assured that the treated area wasn't swelling *too* much, because that could indicate (from their perspective, at least) either an active brain tumor that might need to be treated with radiation or tumor-related swelling that might need to be treated with steroids. Both would preclude me from the trial, as those treatments could throw off their results.

Making matters worse, my latest MRI had shown the treated lesion in my cerebellum had grown from 5.4 millimeters to 8.3 millimeters. Dr. Uhlmann assured me that this growth was normal, and likely represented nothing more than lingering swelling from my Cyberknife treatment about a year earlier.

"So you don't think it's enough to exclude me from the clinical trial?" I asked.

"I think it would be ridiculous if they excluded you for this reason," he said. "A Cyberknife treatment to a healthy brain would show the same kind of swelling, and this is not causing you any problems."

I mentioned Dr. Uhlmann's opinion on my brain swelling to Virginia Seery and Dr. Mier when I saw them later that day to review the terms of the consent form. Their response was slightly less positive.

"Even knowing that, we still have people get turned down," Seery said when I expressed Dr. Uhlmann's take on the matter. "We would make our case—Dr. Mier will go to bat for you, and so will Dr. Uhlmann—but sometimes the medical monitors won't budge."

"Personally, I don't really think you can deliver a dose of radiation to the brain and *not* have swelling," Dr. Mier said. "It's inherent in the way that radiation works. So we're going to ask our radiologists to simply not comment on that unless it's really blatant; that way, it doesn't become an issue."

"Good," I said, while thinking, *I sure hope that's enough.*

"So I gather you're familiar with the side effects of the therapy?" Dr. Mier asked.

I had a copy of the trial information in my lap, thirty-six pages in all, which had been faxed to me at the office the day before. For nivo, the most common side effects appeared to be fatigue, skin problems such as rashes and itchiness, as well as diarrhea, nausea, abdominal pain, joint pain, and fever. For ipi, the top side effect was diarrhea, which seemed to range from mild to very severe with bleeding.

"I don't think you'll feel anything from the nivo," Dr. Mier said. "A few autoimmune side effects, but they're rare. On the other hand, with ipi, the big one there is colitis."

"What's that, exactly?"

"It's a type of diarrhea, like Crohn's disease. Probably not that much different from an infectious source diarrhea, except it's caused by the immune system being turned on," Dr. Mier replied. "People are not accustomed to the thought that their immune system can damage or harm them in some way, but it can. There are lots of diseases that are caused by an overactive immune system, like Crohn's and AIDS."

Dr. Mier explained that the most promising immunotherapy treatments were those that deliberately interfered with the immune system's ability to dial itself down. "The immune system needs to be able to dial itself back to avoid creating autoimmune problems, as we call them. At the same time, the fact that the immune system *can* do that limits how aggressive it can be towards eradicating infection or eradicating a tumor. In our case, we don't *want* those switches activated, we want to stifle them. The resulting side effects are consistent with your immune system getting revved up."

According to the consent form, I would receive both drugs for three months, and my ipi dose would be either one or three milligrams per kilogram of body weight, depending on which arm of the study I was assigned to. All trial participants would receive the same dose of nivo, 3 milligrams per kilogram of body weight.

"I won't know whether I have the larger ipi dose for a while, right?" I asked.

"That's right—not until you've jumped through all the hoops and are on the trial," Seery replied.

"But the lower dose is still considered to be an effective dose?"

"Yes," Dr. Mier said. "They work on similar pathways, but they involve completely separate proteins. The data suggest that they work better together than as single agents. I can't say for sure, but I'm feeling optimistic that this will work."

"So am I," I said, and flashed on my Rube Goldberg immune system getting slightly out of whack, in dire need of an alignment.

● ● ●

Seery called me early Monday morning to let me know that the trial monitors had given me the green light. Luckily, we had decided to err on the side of optimism and schedule my first few treatments on the assumption that I would be admitted. That meant my first infusion was to be the very next day, in room 748 on the seventh floor of the Stoneman Building at Beth Israel.

Driving into Boston with Katharina that hot summer morning, I felt grateful for the privilege of getting access to this trial, as well as once again thankful to my boss, Susan Pikor. She was the one who had provided me with the original referral which had connected me with Dr. Choueiri, and then the talented and devoted team at Beth Israel. I realized how fortunate I was to have access to such top-notch care and to a promising clinical trial.

Now I had to do my part.

My mind kept wandering as we drove the now-familiar route into Boston. *I have to keep fighting this selfish, unpredictable beast wreaking havoc in my body,* I thought. *If I don't, it will keep growing until it ends up killing me—the very host that's been feeding it.*

Maybe the beast and I can coexist. Isn't that likely to be the case anyway? No evidence of disease doesn't mean it's not there—just that a radiologist can't see it on a CT scan.

But even if it's been reduced to a cell or two, clinging to the floor of a remote blood vessel, there's always a chance of a cancer comeback. That would be okay with me, though. Buying even a few years would be just fine.

I squeezed Katharina's hand as we pulled into the Beth Israel parking lot. We headed up the elevator to the seventh floor, where a friendly nurse's assistant named Virginette greeted us at the end of the hall. After weighing me on a scale, she took me to room 748 and readied a bed for me.

A nurse who introduced herself as Tanya bustled into the room. She expertly found a vein in my right forearm—no fear of Dr. Tawa's prodding here—filled three test tubes with my blood, and set an IV line for my first infusion.

About an hour after that, Dr. David McDermott and Virginia Seery came in. They were visiting patients on the floor, most of them participants in various clinical trials who were scheduled to receive infusions. They usually stopped by once the lab had sent up blood test results. Then, if everything looked relatively normal, they signed the drug order that went to the hospital pharmacy, where the drug was made up at the proper dose.

"Well, we know what dose of ipi you're getting," Seery said, as she sat down next to me.

"And?" I asked.

"It's an active dose, but it's lower than the FDA approved dose for the single agent drug," Dr. McDermott said. "The approved dose is three milligrams; you're getting one."

Damn; that doesn't sound like much, I thought. *Wonder if it will still work.*

"There's activity at one milligram too, right?" Katharina asked.

Dr. McDermott nodded. "The whole point of this study is that we're not sure which one of these two combinations—one milligram or three milligrams—is better," he said. "It may take several years to work that out. The bottom line is you're getting the most interesting drug for kidney cancer that we've got at the moment, and you're getting it at an active dose. Whether or not the ipi adds benefit or not is unclear until we try. And you're getting the nivo, which you aren't guaranteed to get in some of the other trials. So regardless, this is a more patient-friendly experience."

"Sounds like this is the one to be in," I said and smiled.

"Yes," Dr. McDermott said, but he didn't return the smile. "The only question is how good it works for you. But we'll give it a try."

The first infusion was the ipi, which took about an hour, as did the nivo infusion that followed. Tanya and Virginette both came by the room several times to check on me and take my vitals—blood pressure, heart rate, temperature—to record for the trial monitors. Both doses were flushed out with saline solution to make sure every precious drop found its way into my veins. When the infusions were finished, Tanya carefully tore the tape off my arm, removed the IV needle, and bandaged my arm.

She sent us on our way with a smile. "We'll see you in two weeks," she said. "Be careful driving home."

My head was swimming a bit, so Katharina drove home. The two doses had made me sleepy. I napped on the ride home, and once we arrived, I rested on the sofa and closed my eyes. I tried to picture my T cells munching on cancer cells, but had a hard time coming up with the images as I soundlessly drifted off into a deep, dreamless sleep.

23 Getting Shrinkage News

"You're in 532. I'll be right over to get your vitals."

I was one of several patients being admitted, having navigated through the Monday morning rush hour maze of construction detours, lane blockages, and backed up traffic to arrive, finally, at the infusion unit on the seventh floor of the Feldberg/Reisman complex at Beth Israel Deaconess Medical Center.

I settled on top of the bed's cover sheets and used the remote to bring myself into a sitting position. I then pulled my laptop from my backpack, powered it up, and started my workday. Heedless of the procedures I was about to undergo, my list of tasks remained extensive; still, I hoped to make some progress on it (if my energy levels cooperated).

I began by writing a press release announcing the hiring of a new Title IX coordinator, but was soon sidetracked by an email from a Boston Globe reporter asking several questions about the pay package of Tony Marx, our previous president. I determined that his query would require the help of the college's chief financial officer to help explain the numbers, and was in the process of sending out a quick email when Tanya, the nurse I'd met during my last visit, entered the room to draw blood.

She carried with her an armful of equipment encased in sealed packaging that she placed next to me on the bed and began unwrapping—first, the hypodermic needle and vacuum tube, then three test tubes for the blood draw, then a square of gauze that she would put beneath my right arm to catch any blood drips. She strapped a tourniquet around my upper arm, gently tapped along my forearm, placed a needle onto the syringe and, with a smooth motion, carefully inserted it into my vein. Success.

She taped the IV line against my arm and quickly inserted first one tube, then the remaining two into the hollow shaft of the syringe. The tubes quickly filled with dark red blood, after which Tanya capped my IV line, gathered the three test tubes, and dumped the small pile of medical waste from my bedside into a bio-waste can in the hospital room. All told, the process took less than five minutes.

"Nice job," I commented.

"You have good veins," she replied. "That helps a lot."

The blood she'd drawn was then sent to the hospital laboratory and reviewed, with special attention being paid to my creatinine and lipase levels. Creatinine levels serve as a proxy for kidney function. For someone with two healthy kidneys, a normal level is between .5 and 1.2. My level was usually in the higher range, about 1.2.

Lipase, on the other hand, is an enzyme associated with pancreas function. One common nivolumab side effect is an increase to lipase levels, which can cause pain. I'd actually experienced this unpleasant side effect after a weekend spent camping out and attending the Boogie and Blues Festival in the White Mountains of New Hampshire. I had only to look at my lipase test results to remind myself that, no matter how enticing a cold keg of Steel Rail beer may be, excessive alcohol consumption and kidney cancer are not good partners. That day, instead of receiving my infusion, I had been sent home. I had since cut back on my drinking, and my lipase levels had returned to normal.

About five minutes after Katharina returned from a quick trip to the restroom, Rose Marujo made an appearance. One of the nurses assigned to clinical trials, Marujo's main responsibility was to work with patients—and the drug companies—to ensure that the trials followed the research protocols that would be required for FDA approval.

"You look kind of uncomfortable there," she said as she entered. "You're lying like you're squished in."

I looked around. "No, I'm fine," I replied. "I'm just getting some work done." *And hoping either you or Virginia has some good news for me.*

The previous Saturday, I had driven into Boston for my scans and I knew that today was the "day of reckoning." The trial protocol called for scans every six weeks for the first three months of the trial. But rather than shrinkage, I had shown slight growth after the first six weeks of infusions. Not enough to kick me off the trial, but definitely enough to worry me that, once again, the immune-drugs weren't working for me.

In his typically optimistic way, Dr. Mier had tried to calm me when delivering my first scan results after commencing the trial. "It could very well be pseudo-progression," he reminded me. "We've seen that in a number of cases, so often that the trial monitors now allow for considerable growth."

My second set of scans, taken six weeks ago, had shown slight shrinkage, enough to kindle my ember of optimism into something more fervent.

I was still continuing with a routine that had served me pretty well so far: my mixed bag of exercise, meditation, guided imagery, and decent nutrition. In other words, both me and my medical team were giving it all we had, and today was the day we found out just how much that added up to.

Problem was, Marujo was clearly not ready to tip her hand.

Instead, she insisted on working through her checklist of questions, trying to tease out any side effects that I might be experiencing from the drugs I was taking. "How's your vision?" she asked. "Any blurriness, waviness or floaters?"

"Not really," I said. "My vision is getting worse, but I don't think it's trial related. It's been going on for a while. I think it's just me getting old."

"Have you been to an eye doctor?"

"Not yet. I've been using reading glasses that I buy at CVS. I had an appointment with an eye doctor about a year ago, but I canceled it. Bigger fish to fry, you know?"

Just then, Virginia Seery walked into the room with a smile on her face.

"Did you tell him yet?" she asked.

"I wanted to wait for you," Marujo replied. "You can tell him, but you can't show him."

By this, Marujo meant that neither she nor Seery could show me the radiologist's actual report. To ensure consistency in the trial, the scans of all clinical trial participants were reviewed by radiologists not affiliated with Beth Israel. I was free to read the reports that Beth Israel radiologists wrote and that the clinic posted online, but that wasn't the report that carried weight with Bristol-Myers Squibb.

"Well, we have the Beth Israel interpretation," Seery said, "and we have the one for the study, which is the one that we technically have to go by. And *that* one says there's been a forty-five percent reduction."

"45.6," Marujo corrected, also smiling now. "Total tumor burden reduction."

"Wow," Katharina, as I sat speechless. "That's...huge."

I was starting to feel very happy indeed.

"You mean all that crap in my lungs and lymph nodes, right? That's the total reduction you're talking about?"

Virginia nodded. "Total reduction means total reduction."

We laughed. Suddenly the atmosphere was almost giddy. We all were beaming.

I asked Marujo why she hadn't let me know as soon as she got in.

"I didn't want to tell you because I knew Virginia wanted to share the good news," Marujo explained.

"Oh, I don't mind," Seery said with a hand wave. "It *is* nice to give good news, though. I've had the opportunity to tell good news a lot lately. I've been enjoying it."

"Does that mean other people in the study are having a good response, too?" I asked.

She nodded, still smiling.

"That's awesome," Katharina said. "That's the best news I've heard in a long time."

"Wow," I said, echoing Katharina. "Just in six weeks? We went from a slight shrinkage last time to this?"

"What we're seeing is, things take a little time," Seery replied. "Even so, we were still happy to see that slight shrinkage last time."

Marujo went back to her checklist and Seery joined the conversation, watching me closely and listening intently to my answers. This was where they started probing about side effects, and whether they were serious enough to warrant action, including stopping treatment.

"Any chest pain?" Marujo asked.

"A little bit of chest pain, but it's probably the immune system killing cancer cells," I said, visualizing the image as best I could.

"What about chills, anything like that?"

I thought for a moment. "Sometimes after coming home from work at the end of a long day I'll get chilly," I admitted.

"But nothing like HDIL-2 though, right?"

"Not like the rigors from HDIL-2, but I still need a couple of blankets. And after a treatment I get kind of cold for a few days."

"How long has that been going on?" Seery asked.

"It just started recently," I said. "But the weather *has* been chilly lately and we don't keep the house that heated to begin with. That said, we have been cranking up the wood stove recently."

Dr. McDermott poked his head in from the hallway, looking to share in the positive vibes.

"Glad to see you guys," he said in his quiet voice, a hint of a smile tugging at his usually taciturn features. "And glad to hear you got some positive news."

"We are very happy," Katharina replied.

"You two deserve it; you've been hanging in there pretty well."

"I'd like to think so," I said. "But it *was* getting a little tense there. Have you been seeing good results with some of the others?"

"Yes, we have," he replied.

"With the combo in particular?"

"Yes, probably the best results are from the nivo/ipi combo."

"What about FDA approval?" I asked.

"We'll have to wait for the results of the trial," he said. "That'll be a while."

Dr. McDermott glanced over my chart briefly, before asking, "And as far as side effects, are you even aware you're on this?"

"Oh, yeah," I said. "I feel fatigued and tired when I come home from work. Mild headaches at times, and I'm not feeling great physically. On the mental side, I've been dealing with anxiety problems, likely due to the uncertainty of everything."

"Well, hopefully these results should help with that," he replied.

"Oh, definitely," I said. "But this has happened so quickly, especially after the slight growth that I had at the beginning of the trial. It looks like the T cells kind of caught on, I guess. Now we can expect maybe a little more shrinkage?"

"I'd say we can, yes. The fact of the matter is there's no documented advantage to an early response. Some of my colleagues actually feel that the people who see the greatest long term benefits are those who take a while to respond initially."

That sounded good to me. "So would you say that I'm about halfway through this trial?"

"Now you're asking for answers we don't really have," Dr. McDermott said. "We're not even sure we've settled on the dose, to tell you the truth."

While Dr. McDermott had been talking, Tanya had come in with the clear plastic bolus bag that contained my dose of nivo and ipi.

"Great news on the scans, huh?" she said, as she flicked gently on the rubber tube, forcing any air bubbles to merge and disappear before the drug entered my veins.

"We're very happy," Katharina said, and I nodded contentedly.

Then it was just Katharina and I, together in an empty room suddenly seemed much less oppressive.

"Hallelujah," Katharina whispered.

"Hallelujah is right," I said. "I'm feeling like fifty might no longer be compressed old age. Maybe I'll get a few more years of life."

"Fifty is pretty young still," Katharina said. "Maybe you can look back in twenty years and talk about this."

In my best "old man" voice, I croaked out, "I had a little bit of a health scare in my late forties, but I came through it okay." It felt good to joke again.

"Maybe you'll beat the odds," Katharina said hopefully.

"Maybe I already am. You don't always beat the odds, and if you do, you don't beat the odds in everything. But I'd rather beat the odds on this clinical trial than win any lottery."

Katharina reached across the bed from the chair she was sitting in and squeezed my hand. We held hands for a while, just soaking up the feeling of contentment. I was learning to savor moments like this. As the bolus bag slowly emptied, I closed my eyes. This time it was easy to picture a Pac-Man-shaped T cell, glowing with extra life as it munched a trail through a mass of dying cancer cells.

24 Full Circle

Flash forward about a year, to an especially busy day for me in Boston—balancing treatment, a hospital visit with a new friend, a brain MRI, and (hopefully) good news from the neurologist.

I had done a decent job of keeping my scanxiety at bay, in part because of an impromptu five-day road trip to the Washington D.C. area. We had perched our bikes on top of our Camry hybrid and motored eight long hours south, through Hartford and the New York City area on our way to suburban Virginia. There, our friends Anna and Dean lived in one of the countless apartment complexes nestled among ribbons of roadway, full to the brim with cars rushing about.

I was lying in our guest bed, trying to sleep off a dinner out with Anna and Dean, when I saw a sudden image in my mind's eye of Steve Baldini.

Baldini and I had met online through SmartPatients and kept in touch through email and the occasional visit. We shared the same cancer, the same medical team, and the same background as HDIL-2 patients. Unlike me, though, he'd been a complete responder, at least for a number of years. His most recent scans, however, had not been encouraging. The Beast had returned, in the form of a sizable tumor in his pancreas.

I reached out for my phone and typed out a quick message:

Hello Steve. How are things? I bet you're glad spring is finally almost here! I have been thinking of you and hoping all is well.

Take care, Peter

The answer came back the next morning:

162

Had surgery yesterday at BI will be here six days I will give you a call when I get home and am feeling better

We wrote back and forth a couple more times. I mentioned I was coming in on Monday and asked whether he was accepting visitors, which he said he was. Come Monday morning I headed to his room, waiting only for Tanya to set up the IV line in my right arm.

By now, I knew the nooks and crannies of the three buildings that make up Beth Israel pretty well, and I also knew the routine of Virginia Seery and the doctors on rotation. They usually came to my floor once the blood lab results were back, a process which took about an hour. They would review the results, ask me about any side effects I was experiencing with the nivo, and sign off on the meds. About an hour later, the treatment would arrive in bolus bags, after which came the infusion, which also lasted about an hour.

All in all, it took from about 9 am to 2 pm for the whole procedure. If everything stayed on schedule, I could just beat the heavy afternoon traffic out of Boston and be back in Keene by 4:30 or so.

I found Steve's room, and we got caught up. Baldini's success with HDIL-2 had been one of the most promising, but just as he was settling into retirement, his life had been thrown into turmoil again. Still, he was facing his situation with courage, stoicism, humor, and a bit of regret that he was going to be missing out on his cigars and red wine, at least for a while.

"You had a good run," I said. "You responded well to HDIL-2, and you were cancer free for more than four years."

"I did have a good run," he agreed. "I did some traveling; even went to Vegas last year. Guy there who gave my wife and I a gondola ride, he asked me the occasion. Told him we'd been married for forty years and that I was a kidney cancer survivor. The guy told me I was looking good, much better than the guy he'd had a week ago. 'That guy had a bucket list and Vegas was on it,' he told me. 'But he didn't look so good. You look good.'"

"I agree with him," I said. "You *do* look good.

"I think about this a lot," I continued. "No matter how bad things get, there is always someone worse off than we are. I feel like I've had a good run, too, all things considered."

My phone vibrated. It was Tanya, calling me back.

"Rose and Virginia are here with your bloodwork," she told me. "They're ready to sign your order but they need to see you first."

I told Tanya I would be right over. Just then, a nutritionist came into the room to go over Baldini's new diet in more detail. With some of his pancreas removed, his fat intake needed to be dramatically curtailed. He wasn't looking forward to it, but he was going to try to be compliant. "If I'd have known I wouldn't be able to eat anything, I don't know if I would have gone through that surgery," he said.

"I don't blame you," I said, giving him a reassuring grin. "Maybe you'll be able to ease up on the diet and cheat every now and then."

"Yeah, maybe I'll hold onto a bottle or two of Bailey's," he mused. "I still have some $30 cigars. I quit smoking when I was diagnosed in 2009, but I've still got quite a collection at home."

"Maybe we can smoke a cigar together to celebrate some good scans down the road," I suggested.

"Let's try to do that," Baldini said. We shook on it and said our goodbyes.

As I walked back to my building I made sure to find the sun in the afternoon sky. Even though it was late March, temperatures were still below freezing. All the same, the sun was strong and warmed my face.

A large gull wheeled above the new Dana-Farber building, and I could make out patients silhouetted inside massive horizontal planks of windows on the upper floors, some of them no doubt looking out at the city—waiting, full of anxiety, for their names to be called.

• • •

Seery and Marujo came in shortly after I'd got myself situated on top of the bed. "You look like you got some color," Seery commented.

"I try to get outside if I can," I joked.

Seery smiled. "So I understand you have a brain MRI later on today?"

"Yeah, it's a busy day," I replied. "I'm trying to get it all done in one trip."

"And how are you feeling?"

"Pretty good," I said. "I'm not really worried about the MRI. I've been able to think about other things and just live day to day."

"I know that's not always easy. Your labs look excellent, by the way."

"That's good. Maybe that's a good sign for the MRI."

"We'll hope so," was all she said.

Dr. Rupal Bhatt, one of the members of the Beth Israel oncology team, entered the room, her lab coat tastefully accented by a colorful swirl of a scarf wrapped neatly around her neck. She smiled and greeted me, before saying, "Your labs look exquisite."

"Exquisite! That's not a word that gets associated with labs very often," I said.

"All the counts look great," she said. "There's nothing out of the normal range."

"That *is* good news." I shot a glance at Seery. "Another good sign for my brain MRI."

Dr. Bhatt smiled with empathy. "We'll be wishing you good luck on that."

• • •

About an hour later (after a bolus bag containing 280 milligrams of nivo had emptied itself into my bloodstream) I made my way back to the Farr building, where my brain MRI was to take place.

Once there, I wandered around a warren of hallways until I found the MRI reception area in a remote corner of the basement. I donned my two-part robe and sat in the chair, filling out my intake questionnaire while workers hauled ladders and tools into the hallway.

The machine itself was situated in a mobile trailer that had been connected to the edge of the building. The radiology attendant led me to a floor lift, and with the press of a button, we slowly rose until we were even with the entrance to the trailer.

MRIs were routine for me by now, and so I settled on my back, my head wedged into what felt like a cushioned vise, breathing slowly and deeply to override the feeling of being constrained that tugged at my subconscious.

About forty-five minutes later, with the loud throbs, drums, and buzzes of the machine still ringing in my ears, I walked back to the eighth floor of the Shapiro building for my appointment with Dr. Uhlmann.

A nurse led to me an examining room, saying the doctor would be right in. I sat waiting for about fifteen minutes, all the while thinking to myself, *This can't be good. He's probably going through the scans and saw something.*

No, that's not it, my optimistic side said. *He's just having a busy day and he's backed up a bit. It takes time to look at all those images.*

My speculation was ended with the arrival of Dr. Uhlmann himself, who gently shut the door and sat down in the chair next to me.

"We looked at the images," he began, "and compared them to the ones we took three months ago. We can see the treated spots; one on the left frontal and the right frontal, so there's two in the front, plus the one on the left side that was also treated.

"Then, there's a new one. This one's tiny, so tiny I can barely see it. It's like the size of a grain of rice. It's on the right side, more towards the back."

The optimism I had worked so hard to cultivate over the past few months dissipated in an instant. "It's in a totally different spot?"

"It's totally different, which is why I think it's real," Dr. Uhlmann confirmed. "I don't expect this to give you any problems; it's way too small for that. On the other hand, I *do* think it will grow unless we zap it, so…Cyberknife would be my recommendation. I'll confer with Dr. Mahadevan; we'll see what he has to say."

"I guess that means the nivo isn't working in the brain?" I asked.

"Well, we don't really know that," he said. "It could be that it is working and things would be worse if you weren't getting that treatment. How were your last scans?"

"They showed that I'm cancer-free from the neck down," I replied. "How often can we really use the Cyberknife? Is there a limit?"

"Well, the thing about the Cyberknife is that while it *is* a very high dose of radiation, as long as the tumor is small, you can handle it. Imagine the radiation you're receiving is something very heavy; lead, for example. You can easily carry a piece of lead the size of a small pebble, but it gets heavier as the size of the lead increases. If you had more tumors, or if they were larger, then we would have to go to whole brain radiation. But that's not called for just yet."

Dr. Mahadevan confirmed much of what Dr. Uhlmann had told me and outlined my situation. "We always knew that there could be microscopic spots that could be seeded later," he explained, "and we talked about whole brain radiation, which we thought would be too much. Now we have these spots which we treated, which look very good, and a new one, which is very small and which we think should Cyberknife."

"Dr. Uhlmann said there'd be no issues with using the Cyberknife again; is that right?"

"As long as they're small, you can be treated again," he said, echoing Dr. Uhlmann's earlier explanation. "Though if they keep coming or start showing up with greater frequency, we would consider whole brain radiation. There's a higher likelihood of neurological side effects from that, and there's no guarantee that the tumors wouldn't come back afterwards."

In the end, we agreed that the Cyberknife was the way to go. The drive back to Keene was extremely lonely. Part of me didn't want to share the news of this latest setback with Katharina, while part of me needed time to come to grips with and accept that cancer was still figuring out ways to gain a foothold in my body.

It could be worse, I reminded myself.

But it could be better, too.

Still, I didn't feel quite as disappointed as I had when receiving bad health news in previous months. Maybe I had become mentally stronger and had learned how to accept my situation. Or maybe I realized that I had already beaten the odds by being in reasonably good shape four years after being diagnosed with Stage IV kidney cancer.

It could even be that I felt less worried about dealing with this latest setback because I wasn't working any more. I had decided to leave my job at Amherst College after almost four years as a Stage IV cancer patient. It had been a tough choice, one that required hours of weighing the pros and cons over and over again in my head, but in the end it boiled down to this: my job had grown less enjoyable and more stressful, even as I experienced increasingly noticeable side effects. I was missing a day of work every two weeks and felt sluggish for at least a day or two after treatment. Sometimes I would feel fatigued for days.

Meanwhile, there was talk of reorganization, a revamped job description, a new boss, and turnover in departments across the college. Even had I not been fighting cancer, it would probably have been time for a change. I did seriously consider two overtures, one from a respected university in upstate New York and the other from an elite private university in the Boston area. I declined both because of my health situation. I had finally accepted that cancer was impeding my professional viability, at least for now.

The immunotherapy *had* truly worked wonders—from the neck down, at least. Still, I couldn't avoid the fact that it was becoming harder to work at the level I and others at the college expected of me. Something had to give, and that something, for now, at least, would have to be my professional life.

My last day of full time work was in late September 2014. It was an abrupt transition—a self-imposed retirement in a way—without much in the way of a plan other than to focus on healing. There were plenty of times in the days and weeks that followed when I'd feel restless, bored and missing my old job. But then I remembered those stressful moments. Maybe early retirement, disability, or whatever I ended up calling it wouldn't be so bad after all. I hadn't asked for it, but why not accept it and make the best of it?

In the weeks that followed my decision to quit working, I had been quickly approved for Social Security disability in an expedited process because of my Stage IV cancer diagnosis. I was also approved for a personal disability policy from Northwestern Mutual that I had been paying premiums on for years. A few months later, the company handling the college's long-term disability policy approved my claim, as well.

It all added up to pay that didn't come close to matching what I had been earning at Amherst, but which still allowed us to meet our living expenses. I would also have my health insurance from work for a couple more years, thanks to federal COBRA legislation. What would happen after that would depend on my health—Medicare, Obamacare, maybe even insurance from another job, if I was healthy enough to be able to work again.

That was down the road, though. For now, I had coverage, and I knew how lucky I was to have it.

By living within our means over the years, Katharina and I had been able to pay our house off *and* cover college expenses for both Max and Jakob, who would graduate within a few weeks.

As I drove home I pictured Jakob, quietly proud in his black cap and gown on Graduation Day at the University of Vermont. It would be a big day, one I had pictured many times over the past few years.

Beyond that, there were plenty of other tasks to take on, energy permitting. Not a bucket list exactly, but a way to find purpose at age fifty in a life that hadn't turned out the way I had envisioned it, but which also wasn't nearly as bad as it could be.

Thanks to modern medicine, exercise, meditation, and visualization, as well as the unflagging support of friends, family, and supportive colleagues, I was still taming the Beast (or trying to, at least) while also accepting my situation…most of the time.

I took the exit off Route 2 and headed north toward Keene. It was time. I took a deep breath and dialed Katharina's number. When she answered, I told her the latest news. My voice didn't waver, though my eyes misted up. When we said goodbye to each other, I focused on breathing deeply as I made my home.

But as it was wont, my mind soon started wandering again.

We've been through worse. We'll get through this, too.

I imagined an army of T cells squeezing themselves through tiny fissures in my blood-brain barrier and munching away on the cancer cells hiding deep within the crevices of my brain. In a few days, the Cyberknife's radiation beam would be aimed at those very same cells. This could very well spur an even stronger immune response. Maybe it would clear up the cancer cells forever. It was a lot to hope for.

Still, why couldn't it be true?

Epilogue
Catching up with Freeman

It had been almost two years since I'd had my last brain tumor zapped, and one year since my last visit with Gordon Freeman, the esteemed immunologist and cancer researcher at Dana-Farber.

On this blustery fall day, I was using a cane, hoping that the reason for my recent limp and soreness in my thigh was a result of tendon and tissue strain, and not evidence of new cancer or complications from recent treatment. Just ten weeks earlier, I'd had both surgery and radiation in connection to that spot in my right femur that had been identified and radiated just over five years earlier. A few cancer cells had apparently survived that blast and been evading those charged-up T cells. The lesion had begun growing again—and causing me pain.

My reason for visiting Freeman was to get caught up on recent developments in the field of immunotherapy, to see whether it was living up to the hype. My main question was this: was there more reason for hope among cancer patients like me, who are trying to buy time against a disease that can strike quickly and at any time?

I stepped out of the elevator and once again walked down the hallway to Freeman's office, which was located near the laboratory where Freeman had conceived of and conducted the research that eventually led to current cancer immunotherapy treatments such as nivolumab. Since then, Freeman had been mentioned in media coverage as being on the short list for a Nobel Prize.

Freeman's door was closed, so I knocked lightly. He opened the door with a smile and welcomed me into his office. It looked

171

as though he had been eating lunch; a sandwich rested on a square of brown wrapping paper on a desk piled high with papers and scientific journals. He motioned me into a chair and asked how I was doing.

Pointing to my cane, I told him my leg was still recuperating from a surgery earlier that summer that involved embedding a metal plate onto the bone using six gnarly-looking metal screws. Eight radiation sessions had followed the surgery, and the healing had been going fine…until I had decided to go for a sail and then a hike. While I *had* been cleared to resume full activity, once again, I had overdone it. The leg hadn't been the same since that active weekend, and I was getting worried. "It's been pretty sore lately, and it doesn't seem to be getting better," I said. "I'm starting to wonder whether I should get it looked at."

"Another chapter for your book, perhaps?" he suggested.

I shrugged. "Maybe," I said. "We'll see."

The truth was that focusing on my own story was draining. It took a lot of energy to remember and write about my past treatments—energy I often felt could be better spent in the moment, rather than dwelling in the past.

I steered the conversation toward Freeman, asking him to reflect on the past year.

"Since we last spoke," I said, "are you surprised that nivo—and immunotherapy in general—seems to have done so well and performed so well in various clinical trials?"

"Am I surprised?" he replied. "No. We had a period when we thought of cancer as one disease, and we've since entered a period where we think of cancer as 200 diseases. But to the immune system, cancer is still more like one disease. The immune system is more concerned with how many targets in the cancerous cell it can attack."

"If the immune system recognizes the cancer cells to begin with," I added as a caveat, keeping in mind the infuriating ability of so many cancer cells to evade detection by the various white blood cells circulating within our bodies.

He nodded in agreement. "On the other hand, there are some tumors that have lots of changes—lots of mutations—like melanoma and lung cancer. Those changes make them good targets for immune therapy. That's been a critical realization.

"The thing about a lot of the old cancer drugs is they hit just one target," he continued. "But if you hit just one target, all the little varieties in the cancer cell let it find a way around the attack. You do well for a year, maybe more, but then it becomes resistant and stops working, all because that one in a billion cancer cell found a way around it.

"What's good about the immune response is you've got millions of T cell receptors and millions of different B-cell receptors, not to mention hundreds of what are called pattern recognition molecules. You've got an evolving system that can change as the tumor changes. You're not a one-trick pony." He paused and added, "But yes, there are certain tumors which are less suited to immunotherapy, like prostate cancer. That's a tough one, because there are fewer changes in the tumor."

My own cancer came to mind, and I briefly pictured the network of tiny nephrons in the kidneys that filter and circulate fluids into the bloodstream. Little wonder, then, that kidney cancer can spread so widely, going from the bones to lymph nodes to the brain.

"In your opinion, where are we now with immunotherapy?" I asked.

Freeman didn't hesitate. "Right now, we're at the monotherapy stage—therapy with one of the immunotherapy agents. I'd say we're at the dawn of combination therapy; things like PD-1 plus CTLA-4 is now an approved drug in melanoma and is being tested in many other situations with success.

"The problem with that nivo–ipi combo is that it's more toxic and requires a lot more medical management to deal with the large number of adverse events," he added. "We're still trying to find the right combination, one that is effective *and* safe. There are more than 800 clinical trials looking at immunotherapy agents, both singly or together with other agents. There's an amazing amount of effort going into finding what works and is safe."

"You certainly seem optimistic," I noted. "But are there any challenges or things that you're worried about in the broad area of immunotherapy? Whether it be on the business side, the research side, the funding side, or the cost side for the patients?"

He paused as he considered the question. "Immunotherapy becoming overhyped is a concern," he began. "Right now, immunotherapy is showing about a twenty percent response rate. A response, in this case, means your tumor shrinks more than thirty percent. It doesn't mean your tumor disappears or you're totally cured. Now, of those, the percentage of people who have a tumor that shrinks 100 percent or ninety-eight percent, that's less than that twenty percent. It's a subset of that. You don't want to overhype things; that leads to unrealistic expectations and negative press for the field."

"One of the big questions, then, is how to get these immune therapies to work for a larger number of people," I summarized. "Where are we at with that? Is that work that is going on at your level, in the lab? Or is it more at the clinical level?"

"It's both," Freeman said. "To put a therapy into clinical trial, you need logic and justification. That's provided by scientists in the lab doing model experiments, usually in a mouse, and finding the agents that work under those conditions. Then you have to test and see if it's safe in something like a monkey. If it doesn't cause damage and isn't inherently dangerous, then you bring that combination to people to see if it's safe. That's always the purpose of a Phase 1 trial. If it's a really effective drug, you may see some efficacy results in that Phase 1 trial."

I thought back to my own experience in a Phase 1 trial. In my case, the trial had tested the combination of nivo and ipi, one of the first times those two had ever been used together. I had definitely experienced side effects, including joint pain that seemed to be getting more severe.[4] I suppose I'm a decent example of the promise

---

4 Since this conversation with Freeman, I've had to stop taking nivolumab because of the severity of arthritis symptoms. Arthritis is an autoimmune response, which means the treatments for it will tamp down my immune system – hopefully not enough to allow the cancer to make a comeback. You better believe I'm working on some new visualization exercises that incorporate this latest twist.

as well as the limitations of immunotherapies. I've responded very well in the lung and the lymph nodes; less so in the brain and my right femur. It was with this mixed success in mind that I brought up my next question.

"I know it's still relatively early to use the word 'cure' for immunotherapy," I said. "There are durable long-term responses, for sure. But I'm wondering what your thoughts are for when someone can be considered cured of cancer, especially Stage IV cancer?"

Unexpectedly, Freeman deflected my question back at me. "How many years do you think are necessary to call something a cure?" he asked. "What do you think needs to be done to establish that you've got a cure? Is it five-year survival? Ten-year? Twenty-year?"

"What do I think?" I asked, thinking, *Why ask me? I'm the patient, not the expert.* "I don't know. It's just such an important word. Is there an accepted medical definition?"

Turning his laptop to face me, he indicated a series of graphs on the display. "This shows the data for over 2,000 patients treated with CTLA-4 since the mid-1990s. Some of these patients have been followed out as long as ten years," he explained, as he pointed to various bars on the graph. "What it shows for CTLA-4 (ipi) is that seventy to eighty percent of people don't do well. But when you get out to three years, the data shows that you're likely to be okay at year four, five, six, seven, eight, nine, ten."

He typed some more, and a new graph appeared on the screen.

"This is a more recent study of around 100 melanoma patients on PD-1 (nivo)," he continued. "PD-1 does somewhat better than the CTLA-4; about thirty-five percent of people are still doing well at five years. The numbers are smaller—the study hasn't been going on as long—but it looks good."

This was all very encouraging, at least for the people who responded to treatment. "Do you have any theories as to why the response rates are still so generally low?" I asked.

Increasing response rates has long been the Holy Grail of cancer treatments, and the quest has proven to be maddeningly elusive. Freeman mentioned that his son Sam was working on the challenge as a PhD student in the Bioinformatics and Integrative Genomics (or BIG) program at Harvard.

"He's actually been looking at kidney cancer," Freeman continued, shooting me a knowing look. "It turns out there's a wonderful consortium called the TCGA, which is a tumor genome atlas. It takes the sequencing information of thousands and thousands of people's tumors, as well as normal kidneys, and puts them into a database that anybody can look at. The idea is to bring all the available data together so that everybody can look at it, use it, and analyze it."

My head was starting to spin—I'm a patient, not a medical expert. That said, I have a sense of curiosity that often overwhelms me if I'm not careful. This was one of those times. "Has he had any interesting findings?" I asked, trying not to sound too excited.

Freeman pulled up another image on his computer screen, this time an image of a kidney. "What the data shows is that kidney tumors—or a lot of them, at least—are very inflamed. What this means is that there's an immune system response going on. The challenge is to make that immune response effective."

"In my case, after I was diagnosed they took out my right kidney and then operated on my left arm, radiating both the arm and my right femur," I said. "They didn't see anything in the early scans in the lungs and lymph nodes. I can even remember Dr. Choueiri saying there was no clinical data to suggest that starting Sutent, for example, would be effective. Do you think we'll get to the point where you would be able to take immunotherapy or some other vaccine as a preventive measure to keep cancer from happening in the first place?"

"I don't think it would be a good idea to try to take immunotherapy before developing cancer," Freeman said. "They're not perfectly safe. The immune system pathways in your body are there for a reason."

"I remember you mentioning that the last time we talked," I said. "You said you wouldn't want your immune system revved up all the time. You want it to stand down after it deals with the threat at hand."

Freeman nodded. "Now, I have a question for you," he added. "The other thing that physicians are studying is, what is a patient's quality of life on immunotherapy as compared to, say, chemotherapy? When you talk to me about biking and hiking and doing these physical activities, that all sounds good to me."

"It definitely is," I agreed. "I do spend a lot of time coming and going from treatment and doing different things related to the treatment. And sometimes the side effects are pretty bad—I get tired for days, and I can get feverish at times. It helps that I'm not working at the moment. It would be hard for me at this point, given how many hours I have to devote to treatment. But my eventual goal is to step back into the work world, if my health allows."

"Is your financial situation okay?" Freeman asked.

"It's okay," I replied, "provided I continue to receive the disability that I get not only for Social Security but through my previous job's long-term disability policy. My insurance will expire in March, and I'll be transitioning over to Medicare to make sure that I can still get coverage for all the treatment that I'm getting."

Freeman eyed me through his glasses with an appraising glance that was not devoid of empathy.

"Cancer has taught me not to worry too much about things and to just accept things as they occur. I've learned not to let myself feel defeated," I continued. "Research can deal with things as they come up, but you can't control everything. I've learned that when you get diagnosed with cancer, there's more out of your control than you'd have ever thought possible."

I stopped talking then, feeling uncomfortable about having shared so much. I felt like I had already taken up too much of Freeman's valuable time.

"Listen," I began. "It's getting to be afternoon, so..."

"You've got important things to do?" he asked with a smile.

I laughed. "Actually, I was thinking that *you* did. I just have my treatment."

"That *is* important," he protested. "I just have to get my glasses from the optometrist."

"That's important, too," I said.

I stood up, we shook hands, and went our separate ways.

I slowly walked the block back from Dana-Farber to Beth Israel. Other pedestrians seemed to glide smoothly around me, going so quickly compared to my slow hobble. I crept toward my goal, leaning on my cane more with each painful step. Just as I had the last time we had spoken, I felt gratitude that someone with Freeman's rare combination of curiosity, intellect, persistence, and ambition was doing his best to move the needle on curing cancer.

But as always, my mind shifted gears to more practical matters. *I better get this leg looked at. That bone may be broken.* The prospect of another long recuperation made me wobble. Still, I caught myself and brightened up, at least for a moment. *If it is broken, then those T cells can get deeper inside,* I thought as I made my way forward. *Then they can kill those cancer cells, once and for fucking all.*

I had a long way to go to reach my appointment at Beth Israel, and each step seemed to take more effort. But I could visualize my destination so clearly. As I've said, I've always been good at working around obstacles, and I'm not one to throw in the towel while there's still hope.

And I wasn't ready to give up yet.

Acknowledgments

It has not been easy to write this book, and it would not have happened without the support and encouragement of many people along the way.

I want to especially thank my wife Katharina for her unstinting support, both as a wife and as a caregiver. My sons, Max and Jakob, have helped me and provided me with more motivation and inspiration than they may realize.

I thank all my healthcare providers, from the oncologists to the nurses, especially Virginia Seery, CRNP, MSN, at Beth Israel Deaconess Medical Center in Boston. She is the epitome of caring, competence and compassion.

The process of researching and writing this book was fairly long and drawn out, in part because of my own health issues. My thanks to Ilan Stavans, Dan Barbezat and Lisa Stoffer at Amherst College, who offered crucial early encouragement, and my indefatigable agent Dede Cummings who found the right publisher.

At Hatherleigh Press, I am especially thankful to Ryan Kennedy for his insightful and meticulous editing and to Ryan Tumambing and Anna Krusinski for their support.

The list of family and friends who have offered their support to me and my family is a long one. Thanks to my parents, John and Ulli Rooney; my siblings and their spouses, John Paul and Linda, Kati and Jim, Anna and Billy David and Julia; my cousins (including Kate and Seth, Sean and Judy, Moria, Ellen, Charles, Matthias and Phil), aunts and uncles (Kath and Doug, Jimmy and Carol, William Driscoll), who kept my spirits up; Katharina's family in Austria, especially Gertrude; and friends, especially Christina and Bob Furlone, Klaus and Christine Bayr, Janice

Warren and Steve Shriner, Anna and Dean Guatieri, John and Marianne McGauley, Beth and Joe Bergman, Bill Watson and Suzanne Welch, Mark Bromley, Anne Mullett, Chris Fox, John Meehan, Hilary Rooney, Ann Nguyen, and so many supportive members of the Spofford Yacht Club, where I hope to return to Sunfish racing some time soon.

About the Author

Peter Rooney has more than a decade's experience working as an award-winning journalist for the Associated Press in Berlin and newspapers in Illinois, where his reporting contributed to the exoneration and release of a death row inmate, and was the subject of his first book *Die Free*. Peter was also vice president at Gehrung Associates, where he helped academic institutions tell their stories through the publication of research breakthroughs, unconventional wisdom from the 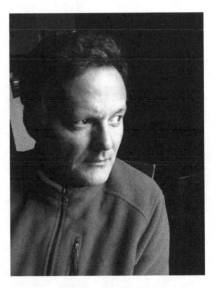 social sciences, and other insights from academia. He was heading up communications at Amherst College when he was diagnosed with advanced stage kidney cancer, which eventually progressed to his bones, lungs, lymph nodes and brain. He met his wife, Katharina, during a year he spent studying abroad in Vienna, Austria, and has two adult sons, Max and Jakob. He lives in Keene, NH.